W9-DGD-080

Identity, Health and Women

# Identity, Health and Women

## A Critical Social Psychological Perspective

Jacqueline Ann Christodoulou
*Ph.D., CPsychol.*

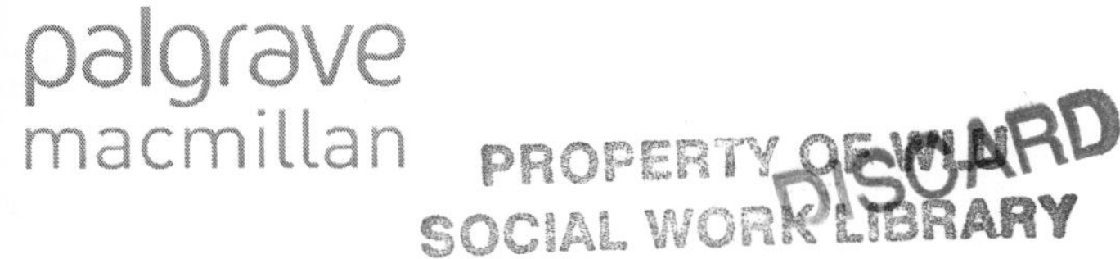

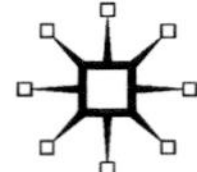



First published 2010 by
PALGRAVE MACMILLAN

Palgrave Macmillan in the UK is an imprint of Macmillan Publishers Limited, registered in England, company number 785998, of Houndmills, Basingstoke, Hampshire RG21 6XS.

Palgrave Macmillan in the US is a division of St Martin's Press LLC, 175 Fifth Avenue, New York, NY 10010.

Palgrave Macmillan is the global academic imprint of the above companies and has companies and representatives throughout the world.

Palgrave® and Macmillan® are registered trademarks in the United States, the United Kingdom, Europe and other countries

ISBN 978-0-230-24179-4 hardback

This book is printed on paper suitable for recycling and made from fully managed and sustained forest sources. Logging, pulping and manufacturing processes are expected to conform to the environmental regulations of the country of origin.

A catalogue record for this book is available from the British Library.

Library of Congress Cataloging-in-Publication Data
Christodoulou, Jacqueline Ann, 1961–
Identity, health and women : a critical social psychological perspective / Jacqueline Ann Christodoulou.
p. cm.
ISBN 978-0-230-24179-4 (hardback)
1. Women–Health and hygiene–Psychological aspects.
2. Women–Health and hygiene–Social aspects. 3. Women–Identity.
I. Title.

RA564.85.C487 2010
613'.04244–dc22 2010027509

10 9 8 7 6 5 4 3 2 1
19 18 17 16 15 14 13 12 11 10

Printed and bound in Great Britain by
CPI Antony Rowe, Chippenham and Eastbourne

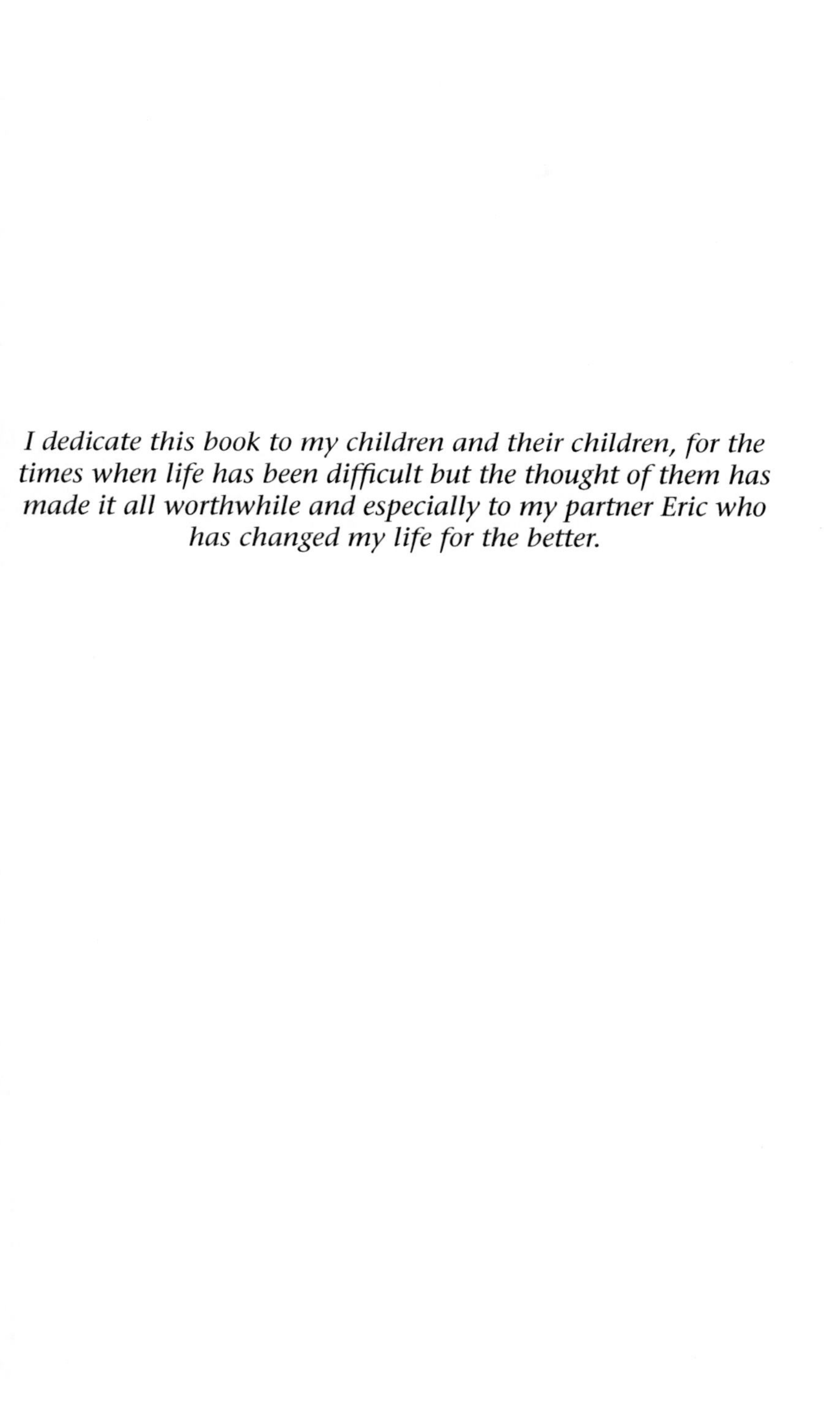

*I dedicate this book to my children and their children, for the times when life has been difficult but the thought of them has made it all worthwhile and especially to my partner Eric who has changed my life for the better.*

# Contents

# List of Figures

# Foreword

This book presents a qualitative exploration of the ways in which perimenopausal women construct and re-construct their health identity. A reflexive approach to the research grounds this study in the North West of England, in a socially and economically deprived regeneration area in the UK. This enables the voices of previously unheard women to shine through the research in a person-centred account of health identity construction.

Using a narrative approach underpinned by a feminist critical realist philosophy, 32 women between the ages of 35 and 55 were interviewed. The interviews were transcribed and analysed in line with Crossley's (2000a) and McAdam's (1993) methodological framework that involves the study of tones and images in the narrative accounts. In addition, a thematic analysis was undertaken to explore issues across all women participants. This was to ground the accounts of the women in societal meanings of femininity, sexuality and family life, linking the personal and the social aspects of identity construction.

The research has identified two key discourses used by these women in their considerations of health – a medical discourse and a relational discourse and shows how the women navigate between these two often competing discourses as their thoughts, feelings and intentions vacillate throughout their health experiences. Additionally, the research shows that women often consider reproductive health from a pathological perspective, yet acknowledge its status of paramount importance in the construction of health identity.

Reproductive milestones such as menstruation, childbirth and menopause operate as narrative touchstones for the explanation of the health narrative. The embodiment of these touchstones in the world is explored through personal, interpersonal, positional and ideological tones, themes and images throughout the accounts, drawing heavily on Murray's (2000) work. Additionally, themes of health strategising were explored which revealed the importance of both wellbeing and illness in social constructions of health identity.

In this book, health identity is situated as a fluid and flexible evolving construction in conjunction with realist considerations of the physiological body. A model of the fluid yet fragmented nature of perimenopausal identity is presented whereby the personal, interpersonal and ideological domains of health, are usefully integrated by the author in an holistic explanation of perimenopausal health experience. The implications of this model for women's health and identity is wide ranging, providing material for the engagement of academics and health professionals in debates concerning the ways in which women are oppressed within service environments and changes that must be made to institute more effective health services. As such, this book is of interest to students and health practitioners alike.

Judith Sixsmith

# Acknowledgements

A large number of people have contributed to the culmination of this project. Major thanks, more than words can express, go to the women who took part in the study that underpins this work. Their voices added a crucial dimension to a formerly flat, medicalised concept of women's health. Thanks also to the Open University Crowther Fund who supported the research through a grant.

Professor Judith Sixsmith provided academic guidance and personal support in difficult personal times for me and her advice and clarity enhanced the research. Professor Paula Nicolson and Dr Paul Duckett, as well as Dr Rebecca Lawthom, supported the final stages of the research and their critique proved invaluable.

Thanks to the Safety and Reliability Society, particularly Dr Bruce Guy whose inspiration sparked a belief that all this was possible, and Oldham Family Crisis Group who work so hard for the benefit of women's safety. Also, to John Clark of Resurrect Studios in Manchester who allowed us to take over for a couple for hours!

I would also like to thank my children, Michelle, Victoria and Anthony for their love, kindness and support in this undertaking. Also, my parents for recognising early my ability and their guidance towards my goal and my grandparents for their extraordinary love and care. Finally, to Eric, my partner, for his unending patience and support.

# 1
# Introducing Health and Psychology

## Introduction

The idea for the study into perimenopausal health, that is used in this book as evidence for a holistic model of identity construction, originated partly from notions of personal health experiences and partly from knowledge of health psychology. By reading about theories of health psychology it is entirely possible to overlay the theory onto lived experience; this can often produce something additional and conflicting that mirrors available theories of health. Many women feel and express in everyday talk that health is full of situations that include both illness and wellbeing and, although they experience them, they do not fully understand them. For example, the nervous wait for a smear test in the doctors' surgery or the restrictive experience of the maternity ward are aspects of lived experience many women endure without question or understanding. In addition to this, some women's stories of their experience of health and the effects of the community they live in on this experience are not the same as the health experience of their male partner.

In searching for woman-centred accounts of the health lifespan, very few studies are interested in women's health experience in this more temporally based way. Most studies are focused on physiological and medical aspects of women's health from the perspective of the health professional or academic researcher, and do not take into account experience lived over a lifetime. In order to marry health psychology theory with health practice, not just that of health professional but also of those experiencing healthcare provision, it is important to study how women consider their health experiences from their own perspective.

Many women including friends, family and work colleagues, tell stories of health in everyday talk. These are in the form of explanations of physiological health matters and how this material health affects their life and relationships and influences their ongoing health story. These autobiographical accounts of health in everyday talk are important in establishing 'who we are' and 'who we are becoming' in terms of health and conveying that health identity to others in order to form various health relationships. In addition to this, these everyday stories form a running narrative of health experience that provides a plot or storyline to the health story.

Concepts of women's health are embedded in aspects of lived experience from family to spirituality, from childhood to old age. In fact, concepts of health are an integral part of being a person (Marks et al., 2001). The way that one considers health, not only in terms of illness but in terms of also framing wellbeing into the way life is lived, affects all areas of lived experience.

Health is also a highly gendered concept with biological health and the reproductive cycle becoming a natural gender division (Sixsmith & Boneham, 2003). Within this division, it has been argued that, women's health has become objectified through patriarchal social constructions in health provision, science, economics, politics, society and culture (Ussher, 2000; Yardley, 1997). Women's health is often objectively structured around milestones in the reproductive cycle and also forms a continuous psychological sub-narrative that contributes to the construction of the individual woman's health identity. The person she has been, is now and will become is grounded in the status of health enjoyed by the woman that, in turn, influences not only her ability to act on the world, but also her perceived position in society.

In terms of these varying discourses, the perimenopause is an important part of women's health. The perimenopause, a gradual developmental process that spans the time from childbearing years to loss of fertility, is a period where women have experienced some or all of the milestones of the reproductive cycle and experienced other health-related events that have contributed to the construction of a health identity.

The format of this book is an integration of theory and evidence in the form of narrative interviews and ways the analysis of these can inform social change. The women who took part in the study were perimenopausal. Their accumulated health experiences over the lifespan up to the perimenopausal stage have contributed to the demystification of how women construct their health identity. Due to the uniqueness of the health experience over time, women have many different accounts of how health has affected them. A critical realist perspective is taken throughout in order to account for, in addition to socially constructed aspects of women's health, realist notions of the material bodies of women. This underpins a feminist approach to understanding women's lives using feminist standpoint theory that prescribes the investigation of difference within difference. When studying health within this construct, due attention must be paid to the material body as well as direct health experiences to negate a Cartesian dualist model of health.

Research has shown that it is not only direct health experiences that contribute to the internalisation of knowledge about illness and wellbeing (Lyons, 2000; Lyons & Griffin, 2002). Other information such as social representations of health, health relationships and vicariously represented health experiences also contribute to the construction of a health identity. In this book, external representations of health that emerged from the autobiographical accounts of the participants are analysed in order to assess the location of these social representations in relation to women's health. It is pertinent to investigate women's health and identity in the context of both the personal and the social world and evaluate if the dawning of the new postmodern theoretical age is reflected in praxis. The personal health experiences of women today can be elucidated and the theories critically assessed by taking a feminist standpoint in terms of women's experiences to study narrative accounts of women's health. Further, evaluation of these autobiographical accounts in terms of current research and theory in the fields of health psychology, feminist theory and critical realist philosophy, will provide a link between theory and the praxis of these lived experiences. In addition to this, evaluation of the accounts in terms of their location in the social world will provide depth of analysis in terms of clarifying the effect of the politics of women's bodies.

The material in this book is concerned not only with illness as a construction of health, but also with wellbeing. The psychological narrative account of health and identity in this book is investigated through semi-structured interviews. This illustrates how health is embodied in concepts of joy and love in addition to suffering and pain in a woman's life through events such as childbirth and work and how coping strategies that women have used during periods of difficult health have become positive and empowering experiences. In the following sections, an exploration of how health psychology has progressed is detailed so as to clarify the ways in which construction of health can be investigated.

## Deconstructing health – Early notions of health

Health concerns are an integral part of life and the historical and theoretical context of health are investigated in order to evaluate how ontological and epistemological developments have influenced present day thinking (Foucault, 1978). In this book a holistic model of critical health psychology is theorised, and in order to do so, the introduction will point to early models of health and trace the progress of constructions of health and how they have been investigated through centuries until the present day.

In early thinking, theoretical division between the mind and the body were not made and the health issues of illness and wellbeing were often thought to be the result of an element of an external spiritual influence (Ogden, 2000). Hippocrates (circa 377BC) and Gallen (circa 199AD) proposed the theory that four fluids within the body, black and yellow bile, blood and phlegm were responsible for health complaints including psychological illness such as depression and madness and that, conversely, wellbeing was promoted by attention to the condition of these fluids (Taylor, 1999).

Later Descartes (1647, in 1969 translation) furthered the consideration that the mind was a separate entity to the body, otherwise known as Cartesian dualism or the mind/body split. Descartes' argument for mind/body dualism rests heavily on religious faith to determine health and views the body as a mechanical vessel that is controlled by the mind or soul via 'a small gland at the base of the brain' (Descartes, 1647, in 1969 translation, p.18).

Essentially, Cartesian dualism formed a basis for the development of the biological model of medicine that was to emerge out of Darwin's theory of evolution.

During the 18th and 19th centuries, health and illness became almost exclusively biologically based. With the development of new technologies and advances in medicine and medical procedures, progress was made in the cataloguing of symptoms, diseases and remedies, and the medical institution was built on the basis of empirical scientific discoveries using experiments on human bodies. As a result, these empirically tried and tested diagnosis and treatments reinforced the mind/body dualistic model of biological medicine. In this model illness, not wellbeing, was the focus of health. Illness was seen as a body invaded by bacteria or virus or such. This meant that theories of illness were primarily based on cellular change and consequently only medical experts and professionals had the skills and knowledge to deal with health.

Darwin (1859) later proposed the theory of evolution and argued that human beings were evolved through time from the basic elements of nature and were biological in essence. This further reinforced the scientific biological model of health and medicine and the divide between the mind and body in terms of responsibility for ill health and wellness. By naturalisation of the body in scientific terms it was possible to pass the responsibility for diagnosis and cure to the medical profession. As the body was now assumed to be natural in essence, any pathological changes were explained, according to the biomedical model, caused by forces outside the affected person, leaving them as a passive victim of illness (Ogden, 2000). At this point psychological aspects of health were discounted and the material body was still regarded as machine-like. Progress towards a more holistic understanding of health was made with the inclusion of psychological matters in consideration of illness and wellbeing.

## Health and psychology

Developments of psychological theories based on health during the 20th century linked the body with the mind and began to include psychological aspects of health in a cause and effect manner. Psychosomatic medicine was introduced and integrated into the biological model of health, most notably with Freud's psychoanalytic theory of the unconscious mind. Freud's work on hysteria as a psychosomatic condition opened up the field of medicine to include psychological aspects. This important and timely link between health and psychology was the beginning of the discipline of health psychology as a field of study that, taking into account physiological illness, also considered any psychological aspects of health. However, Freud's work has been criticised on the basis of too heavy a reliance on the unconscious mind and the lack of attention to material symptoms of health.

Dunbar (1943) and Alexander's (1950) work on psychosomatic illness highlighted the connection between the mind and the body when considering health. Their work, which considered various psychological responses to illness, also identified physiological auto-responses in the central nervous system to stressful situations. They found that these physiological responses worked in conjunction with the psychological responses and were of equal importance in evaluating health. Considering that psychoanalytic work placed too much focus on the mind and not enough on the body, Dunbar and Alexander attempted to rebalance psychosomatic medicine into a discipline which took into account both material and psychological aspects of health. These early theories formed the basis of the discipline of health psychology which challenged the purely biomedical model as discussed above and points to the biopsychosocial model of health and illness (Engel, 1977).

## Health psychology and social constructions: The biopsychosocial model of health

Engel's (1977) biopsychosocial model of health and illness is comprised of integrated factors of biological, psychological and social causes of health and illness. The inclusion of psychological and social factors was necessary, according to Engel, because the recognition of psychological and social issues such as class difference, employment opportunities and housing are implicated in health inequalities and their effects on health. A movement away from the biomedical model of illness towards a more holistic and multidimensional explanation of the cause of illness was a very important turning point in the development of the discipline of health psychology. Engel's model illustrates how internal psychological and external social factors can contribute to illness and consequently how behavioural factors can influence health. This view in turn underpinned a shift away from the medical profession back to personal responsibility for health-related behaviour.

Building on the development of health psychology, Gatchel et al. (1989) extend the field by including more psychosocial aspects of health. The biology underpinning the physiological bases of health and behaviour and stress, stress management and cardiovascular disorders are considered in this work. In methodological terms the behavioural model of health is discussed and several quantitative studies are presented to illustrate retrospective and prospective work on behavioural health.

This illustrates how, in considering models of health, thinking progressed from the medical and behavioural model to the inclusion of a more psychologically-based model. This step to inclusion of prevention and intervention is an important development towards the acknowledgement of health as a concept that is partially the responsibility of the person experiencing health in that they are decision-makers in jointly caring for their own health. This development of a behavioural-based model for health psychology is expanded by Baum's (1999) paper. Baum states that:

> Research increasingly suggests a strong link between how people think, feel and behave and how well they withstand illness and

> poor health. Stress provides one model for understanding and predicting the impact of more specific emotional arousal and distress. (Baum, 1999, p.4)

Baum also proposes that:

> Psychological processes and emotional states influence the aetiology and progression of disease and contribute to overall host resistance or vulnerability to illness. (Baum, 1999, p.7)

This provides an explanation of how stress in conjunction with risky health behaviour can contribute to the cause and/or pathological progression of chronic illness such as cancer, cardiovascular disease and HIV/AIDS. This is an important consideration as it gives an overview of how lifestyle can affect biology, but unfortunately does not emphasise social factors such as class, gender, poverty levels etc. The methodology of the experiments cited by Baum is mainly quantitative and the theoretic stance is clearly based on the biomedical model with a limited psychological perspective as a starting point, viewing any psychosocial contributions as recent developments. Whilst Baum's work is informative, a qualitative methodology that investigates social, cultural and political aspects of risk taking and health would clarify the impact of external representations of health and allow for the design of interventions based on these.

Ogden's (2000) work widens the field of mainstream health psychology to include studies which are more qualitative in nature. Ogden examines health belief models and illness cognition models providing a useful comparison of different paradigms of health behaviour strategies. A useful example of this is Ogden's overview of work on the inter-relationship between beliefs, behaviour and health using placebo as an example. By examining the effect of placebos on health, a practice that had been carried out for decades, a connection is established between beliefs, behaviour and health which have the following implications for health psychology and mind/body dualism.

Ogden's work on the placebo effect highlights the link between medical constructs of health and psychological constructs of health. The medical model of health as a cure for the body as represented in the administration of drugs (or placebo) and the psychological construct of health as psychosomatic are acknowledged by Ogden, moving away from the biomedical model towards an integrated model which deals with more qualitative and multidimensional emotional aspects of health.

Engel's (1977) biopsychosocial model of health and more recent developments in mainstream health psychology conceptualised that health and illness was not solely biological, but occurred in the context of social and psychological influences (Crossley, 2000a). Engel's model reframed health by combining material physiological health and illness with the health experience from a person-centred perspective and providing an interactive framework for the study of health. This allowed for the social constructions of health experience to be taken into account when considering a person's health situation. As can be seen above, progress made in health psychology has become more inclusive of social and psychological aspects of health that inevitably include socially constructed experience.

Whilst the biopsychosocial model of health appears to be holistic and interactive, the base of positivist thinking remains a strong methodological undercurrent. The socially constructed aspects of the biopsychosocial model have been aligned with the physiological aspects of health and are often investigated in a cause and effect manner. This produces empirically grounded evidence that implies predefined measures such as beliefs and attitudes based on quantitative values on which further investigations are based. An example of this is the Hospital Anxiety and Depression Scale (HADS) (Zigmond & Snaith, 1983). Whilst this progress has been useful in terms of the recognition of social and psychological factors, the methodology, (which is an often quantitatively grounded or mixed method of quantitative and qualitative) can leave the unique health experience in the social context unattended.

Social constructivist theory recognises the location of the self in the personal and social world, in a highly fluid, complex and interactive process of construction of experience (Sapsford, 1987). Social construction of experience involves the impact of society on the personal self in a cumulative and ongoing fashion; as health forms an important area of experience, therefore health experience is included in the social construction of experience (Frank, 2000a). As socially constructed experience is fluid and unique, each person experiences a different perspective, and health experience forms part of experience in general, the quantification of health experience may be unhelpful in this context.

Work carried out since Engel's 1977 model of biopsychosocial health psychology which suggests that mainstream health psychology may still be entrenched in the biomedical model of health, even though it [illegible]ims to integrate the experience of health. This invites the critique [illegible] method of analysis excludes an important aspect of health [illegible] understanding the specific and the unique qualities of health [illegible]xperience from the person-centred perspective. This critique of mainstream health psychology, including the biopsychosocial model, is based on those taken up by critical health psychologists who recognise the need to remove the cause and effect values of quantification of health and include the individual social and cultural lived experiences that impact on a health identity.

## What is critical health psychology?

Critical health psychology aims, as its name implies, to critique mainstream health psychology. Critical health psychologists (for example, Marks et al., 2001) recognise that, in order to study health and indeed to produce a balanced state of health, health must be studied in the context of society, culture, politics, ideology, spirituality and personal experience. Critical health psychology aims to challenge the quantitative values of mainstream health psychology and reframe health in the context of social equality/inequality, political power and oppression. Prilleltensky and Fox (1997) explain this as follows:

> We believe that psychology has the potential to help bring about a significantly better world, in keeping with its ethical mandate to promote human welfare. Yet too often we settle for too little. (Prilleltensky & Fox, 1997, p.3)

Taking mainstream health psychology outside the 'normalised' grounding of scientific and objective Western thinking, this critical model takes as its project social injustice and change as a catalyst for improved health. The biopsychosocial model of health psychology includes psychological and social factors in order to predict the causes and effects of health from a humanistic perspective and to modify behaviour towards wellbeing. A difference between this and critical health psychology is that critical health psychology aims to *understand* psychological and societal influences on health in the context of explicitly ideological and political standpoint and is often oriented towards bringing about changes in the external world to address those inequalities that promote ill health. Additionally, critical psychology works to:

> ...challenge dominant societal values and the institutions that reinforce them for a variety of reasons, in a variety of ways. (Prilleltensky & Fox, 1997, p.4)

So, critical health psychology is a relatively recent approach used to study experience of health concerns and illness in the context of society. On a theoretical level, there are major ontological and epistemological differences between mainstream health psychology and critical health psychology. Ontologically, the focus of what is studied moves from the objective model of the patient in mainstream health psychology to notions of subjectivity in relation to both illness and the concept of wellness. Epistemologically, mainstream health psychology's positivist scientific approach based on the empirical testing of theory is criticised as attempting to be clinical and objective. Critical health psychology, whilst reconstructing the subjective ontology, aims to gather knowledge based on a hermeneutic assessment of experience. Whilst Engel's (1977) biopsychosocial model and consequent developments of this integrated system in health psychology provides a more complex and integrated model than the biomedical model of illness, the integral components are presented as individual and fragmented (Crossley, 2000a). In contrast, and in line with the explicit value position of critical health psychology, human experience of health and illness in general flows in an inherent combination of biological, psychological and socio-cultural experiences (Marks et al., 2001). Marks et al. (2001) describe the state of health as:

> Health is a state of being with physical, cultural, psychosocial, economic and spiritual attributes, not simply the absence of illness. (Marks et al., 2001, p.4)

Further, because of the infinite number of possible combinations of external socio-cultural situations interacting with our internal psychology and biology, each individual experience is unique. It is this uniqueness of experience that, Crossley (2000a) argues, underlies the formation of identity. Expression of meaning through communication on the basis of concepts such as attitude, emotion and feelings are the very centre of the social world, and such discourse is a hermeneutic tool when considering the human perspective of health and illness. Therefore, although the use of qualitative methodology does not necessarily imply a critical approach, qualitative methodologies that involve the study of accounts of health and illness are appropriate ways to critically study health.

Critical health psychology is a sub-division of critical psychology but the basic tenets of critical psychology apply equally to critical health psychology. Prilleltensky and Nelson (2002) recommend some basic values that inform their vision of critical psychology: social justice, self-determination and participation, caring and compassion, health and human diversity. The quest for social justice is important to critical health psychologists as the identification of social injustice in society through the investigation of people's lived experiences is a direct comment on aspects of suffering that can benefit from direct interventions.

Critical psychology is invested in social change and aims to challenge institutional power dynamics in order to action this change. This maps onto a critical health agenda by evaluating health in the light of culture and society, as defined by Marks et al. (2001) above, and also evaluates the context of health, including institutionalised health.

Critical health psychology also has important implications for the mind/body dualism debate. In considering mental health, Crossley (2000a) observes that literature in health psychology rarely mentions mental illness and comments that:

> ...this is because over the last twenty years or so in psychology, the study of mental health and illness has been appropriated mainly by clinical psychology. (Crossley, 2000a, p.104)

Again, knowledge generation in clinical psychology often relies on a positivist model and consequently a symptomology of mental illness based on specialist discourse has constructed a specialist field (Mishler, 1984). This has served to distance the 'mental' or 'mind' away from the physical or bodily aspects of health psychology, reinforcing mind body dualism, which is a recurring theme in mainstream health psychology. This specialist discourse oriented model of clinical psychology includes the social construction of the normal and abnormal in illness (Mishler, 1984). Therefore, a more existential, phenomenological approach to the study of mental illness employing the study of individual accounts of illness will expose the complex biological, psychological and sociocultural context of that experience.

In critically reformulating the study of pain and disease, health psychologists (such as Crossley, 2000a; Frank, 2000a; Marks et al., 2001; Mishler, 1999) have moved away from clinical intervention to preserve health and prolong life at any cost, towards 'living in the face of death' (Crossley, 2000a, p.158). The adherence to mainstream health psychology towards the biopsychosocial model promotes the health/illness linear axis in terms of health being the perceived norm. Critical health psychology suggests that concepts such as acceptance of death and appreciation of life contribute to quality of life in illness and individual accounts of these should be studied to gain insight into the nature of multidimensional health psychology.

## Embodiment in critical health psychology

Yardley (1997) has developed an embodied discourse approach to critical health psychology which takes into account the physical and biological aspects of health. Yardley examines a discursive approach to the meaning of embodied experience and provides useful examples of the way qualitative discursive methods can contribute to the study of physical aspects of life through explanation leading to meaning in context. Yardley explains that this material discursive methodology is an attempt to quash the postmodern 'radical relativism' position where there is no truth (or conversely everything is equally and relatively true). Again, the material body combined with a discursive constructionist element is linked to critical realism (Danermark et al., 2002) where the intransient structure of nature and the body can be combined with the constructed nature of the social world. Whilst this may seem to reinforce the mind/body dichotomy further, the aim of material discourse methodology is to combine social, cultural and political fabric into a holistic integrated model of interaction, with no emphasis on one or the other. This, therefore, furthers a critical approach as it allows for considerations of the embodied nature of health experience as equally important to the inward experience of health as well as external representations of health, thereby providing a link between the two in lived experience. Similarly, Ussher (1997) looks at ways of combining the material and the discursive in the study of health and illness. Ussher questions scientists and clinicians on their:

> ...reliance on realist assumptions, failing to question the social or discursive construction of bodily experience, the influence of their own subjectivity or ideological standpoint on the theories or therapies they develop, and the role of scientific or legal discourse *associated with the body* in social regulation and control. (Ussher, 1997, p.5)

Ussher explores material and discursive elements in the construction of various social situations including health and illness in relation to social control. These are important aspects of critical health psychology and potential interventions towards social change.

Embodiment and the construction of a health identity is the subject of Frank's (2000a) discussion of the body, illness and ethics. Frank provides an applied methodology and analysis, including a detailed in-depth explanation of the material body in terms of illness perception.

Frank describes chronic and terminal illness as a disruption or breakdown of identity and observes 'the commonality of suffering cuts across worlds of race and gender as well as types of disease' (p.170). This observation fits well with critical health psychology's holistic values of compassion, caring and diversity (Prilleltensky and Fox, 1997) as it adds the cross-cultural aspect of suffering to the biopsychosocial model when considering illness. Aspects of power and constraint involved in one's own perception of sickness are explored and Frank explains the expectation of sickness from both the standpoint of the sick person and the medical profession:

> Whether or not the sick role describes the experience of being ill, and most agree it does not, it remains a powerful narrative of what medicine expects from the ill person and what other social institutions expect from medicine. At the core of those expectations is the assumption of restitution: returning the sick person to the status quo ante. (Frank, 2000a, p.83)

Frank's narrative typology is based on accounts of experience, as is much of discursive and narrative methodology. Narrative accounts of experience encompass the past, the present and the future (McAdams, 1993) and many narrative psychologists take a lifespan perspective. An autobiographical account of the life of a person grounds the present context of the account in beliefs and attitudes built up over time and provide an opportunity to understand the current health situation (Greene, 2000a). Additionally, understanding past experiences and how these have impacted on the current account in social context can effect social change in the sense that, past meanings can be re-negotiated and modified. For example, attitudes and beliefs about smoking behaviour may be grounded in past experiences of 'the golden age of cinema' where film stars were often portrayed as glamorous and sophisticated while smoking a cigarette. These attitudes and beliefs are thankfully outdated by social change regarding the health risks of tobacco smoking, but it would be helpful to establish, by taking into account past experiences, as to why smoking behaviour continues.

Therefore, stories built up over time provide a cumulative grounding of experience and a more explanatory basis for ongoing construction of experience, leading to better understanding and maximisation of social change. The stories, inevitably, will include aspects of lived experience in the world and include experience of living in society.

## Health and the social world – The politics of women's health

In order to evaluate the influence of the social world on the construction of women's health identity it is important to understand what kind of influences contribute to the construction of meaning around women. There are many different kinds of issues in society that affect women's sexuality, appearance, behaviour and health. Society dictates and disciplines women (Bartky, 1998) into roles at work, in the family and in health and power dynamics, and politics around women in society impact on the construction of identity. Below are some examples from the social world to illustrate how women are affected on a societal and institutional level.

### Politics and women's bodies

The politics of women's bodies involve a variety of different ways that women are affected by influences in society. These include sexual health and control of fertility, body image, abortion and birth control. The societal and cultural situations of women can have an effect on the way that the politics of women's health and bodies affect their lives. Power dynamics in society that surround the meaning of women's bodies and the potential for individual women to influence decisions made on a macro level by institutions such as the government and the NHS provide a complex living environment for women and their health (Weitz, 1998).

In this book the connection between the politics of women's bodies and health and the way that feminist theory has developed into a vehicle for reform and change is recognised. Investigation of the considerations women take into account when constructing a health identity attempts to deconstruct some of the political effects by considering the personal, interpersonal and ideological aspect of how the women live their everyday health. This has been done by investigating how women's bodies are perceived in the context of health psychology (and consequently medicalised and patholgised) and by interpreting how the women narrate their everyday lived experience. This includes how they are influenced by personal relationships and by institutionalised health in addition to their personal health, illuminating the social and cultural conditions of their politicised health and bodies. It was important to look beyond the personal aspects of health encountered by these women and look to institutional effects that contribute to the power dynamic and hence the politics of women's health.

The economic and political interest in HRT is an example of how issues around women's bodies are politicised. This is often not in the direction of total wellbeing for women but influenced by financial considerations. By promoting HRT as a cure for the menopause and other related health problems, agencies may be placing women further under the control of the medical world by creating a reliance on prescribed drugs and consequently increasing financial benefits for pharmaceutical companies. Also, HRT is not without its risks. In addition to the proposed benefits to health and relief of menopausal symptoms, there is also an increased risk of breast and ovarian cancer associated with the use of HRT. Promotion of HRT by government departments politicises women's bodies holding up the ageing process as pathological, as something that can be cured and by suggesting this cure through NHS funding of HRT. Similarly, with legislation regarding abortion and NHS adherence to laws that influence women's reproductive bodies, institutions present a joint political power that is difficult to resist, especially in the face of deprivation and disadvantage. Often, the negative aspects of medical intervention, influenced by governmental political ideology, is not disclosed and individual women have, in everyday lived experience, only one option presented to them. For example, women who choose abortion are presented as pro-choice decision-makers in charge of their own destiny, but often in deprived communities, abortion is the only option open to them. In this case, their bodies are politicised in line with the power dynamics of a society which remains the focus of a critical agenda.

### Politics and the media

The media is another institution in society where power dynamics are present and affect women in their everyday lives. Role models in the media are often held up to dictate appearance and behaviour (Hardin, 2003). Research into the effects of societal influences on body image is becoming more prevalent as eating disorders such as anorexia nervosa increase. Women's bodies are objectified by Western society's model of what is sexually desirable and through the necessity of sex to reproduce and a corresponding discourse (Jose, 1995). Whilst this does vary from time to time, a general guideline for sexual desirability is modelled around youth, whiteness, and thinness (Conboy et al., 1997).

The effects of this mediation of slender young women can be seen in studies by Cussins (2001), Hardin (2003), Thompson and Stice (2001), Wilcox and Laird (2000) and Williams et al. (2003). These studies investigate the effects of body image disturbance and eating pathology and find that the images of 'super slender' women that the media have are linked with eating disorders such as bulimia and anorexia and affect the mental health of some women. The potential fatal effects of eating disorders, and the effects of the media on these, point out the severity of this problem in society. Hardin (2003) considered discourses of anorexia as presented in published autobiographies of women's accounts of surviving anorexia and from a publicly accessible internet bulletin board anorexia message group. They found that:

> Increased media coverage, made for TV docu-dramas, talk shows, magazines, novels and psychology self-help books have increased the public awareness about the act of self-starvation. By telling and retelling cautionary tales, such as accounts of women who have 'survived' anorexia nervosa, the press wields a double-edged sword – they are turning into an advertisement for that very thing. (Hardin, 2003, p.213)

Again, it was found that media use included scanning cautionary tales of eating disorders for information on 'how to be anorexic'. This shows that representations of women in society can have an effect on health.

This is an example of how women are disciplined towards a prescribed model of femininity by power dynamics. These power dynamics are the politics of women's bodies and how women are empowered or oppressed. In addition to this, the reproductive health of women and the work roles of women closely interact in society in competition with men's work roles. PMS and menopause represent a perceived 'difference' in the ability of women to work outside the home and again a patriarchal society provides a disciplined norm towards which women must strive whilst ignoring the cycles of their body which are perceived as a weakness to be mocked or punished by oppression (De Beauvoir, 1949; Bartky, 1998). This perceived 'difference' is an important factor in identity study as it highlights an area where the politics of oppression are at work and similarities and differences in identification in relationships and society are used as power dynamics. Similarly, the politics of housework, or unpaid work within the home, centre around expectations of women in society to complete unpaid work as duty, whilst men 'do it for us' (Malos, 1995, p.164). Many of these power dynamics are influenced by a woman's social and economic positioning in society.

There are many institutions in society that impact on women's health and influence the construction of women's identity. These include medical organisations, religious organisations, the media and society's constructions of the family. In addition to this, overarching constructs of society such as gender, class and ethnicity also contribute to the formation of identity (Woodward, 2004).

## Politics and everyday living for women – The personal and the social

The examples above of the politics around women's bodies and the influence of the media on women's health are clearly linked in their potential to impact on experiences of health for women. The promotion of HRT and the construction of femininity by the media, and the involvement of social institutions such as the media and the government to influence these ideologies indicate a societal level of health that, in everyday terms, is available to all women who live in society. The examples above show that health can be influenced by societal issues. It is no secret that, in today's UK society, many problems (health and otherwise) encountered in everyday living are political and complex. The next section examines attempts by government agencies to assess and address these societal issues and illustrates how the places women live produce a wider political agenda for health.

## Indices of deprivation

The annual public health report for Oldham, a town in the North West of the UK and where the women who took part in the study live states that this town:

> ...experiences some of the worst health in the UK. The need for health care services and ability to access and make use of them is influenced by deprivation...the borough is the 38th most deprived local authority out of 354 local authorities in England. Three of the wards in the borough are amongst the 1% most deprived wards in the country. (Public Health Report, 2004)

The measurement for the deprivation mentioned in the Public Health Report is sourced from the governmental report 'Department of Environment Transport and the Regions Indices of Deprivation' (IMD 2004). This report devises a way of measuring the disadvantage and deprivation of communities by taking societal factors, which are problematic, measuring these, and interpreting them using factor analysis. This produces a ranked table of communities that shows where the most and least problems of deprivation lie.

The Indices of Deprivation originated in 2000 when the office of the Deputy Prime Minister became responsible for regeneration issues in England and Wales. In order to fund regeneration, including improvements to health, the government needed a way to measure which communities needed regeneration most. To do this, the government set up a regeneration unit to collect data from communities about problematic social issues. These were divided into seven domains of deprivation: income deprivation; employment deprivation; health deprivation and disability; education skills and training deprivation; barriers to housing and services; living environment deprivation; and crime. This information was then combined into an index of multiple deprivation using factor analysis. The statistics produced by this are used to measure the deprivation of a community and considered in decisions involving regeneration funding.

The decisions made about community funding occur at government departmental level, and the current government fund regeneration in the most deprived areas as indicated by the indices of deprivation report. The domains in the report are described as interactive indicator of deprivation and include health as an indicator for deprivation on community levels. Everyday living in community settings is therefore politicised within society by levels of deprivation being set and decision-making about addressing deprivation being made at government level.

As the report above mentions, the focal town in this study is measured as the 38$^{th}$ most deprived of 354 towns and boroughs in England at the time of the study, falling to 34$^{th}$ in 2007. Much of the town is undergoing regeneration through government funding and this filters through to the community as new-build services such as health and community centres and health improvement schemes. This may seem an ideal model for a positive critical agenda, where core needs such as social injustice, oppression and valuing diversity are being addressed and this may be the aim of the government departments that designed the Indices of Deprivation and regeneration programmes. Despite this, the regeneration initiatives have subsequently received heavy criticism. This was due to reports of alleged misappropriation of funding and staffing of projects by bringing in staff to highly paid regeneration posts from outside the deprived area and therefore not generating employment for the deprived area. Slow planning of new build projects and poor location planning so as not to include minority groups have also been highlighted (Ritchie, 2001). These critiques of political aspects of community building were widely publicised in the local press. Because of this media coverage, in addition to living conditions experienced, the community was further disparaged by power dynamics that were out of their control through lack of local individual voices within the regeneration decision-making process.

By labelling Oldham as deprived, the lives of individual women in the area are being affected by creating the conditions for a pessimistic political climate. The Public Health Report for 2004 states that the town:

> ...is one of the areas that have life expectancy at birth that is in the bottom 20% of life expectancy across the country...residents have a shorter life expectancy than their counterparts living in Greater Manchester, The North West Region and England and Wales as whole. (Public Health Report, 2004)

Hidden in the domains of deprivation are implications for deprivation that particularly affect women such as low income, poor childcare, single parenthood, teenage pregnancy and poor health services (Sixsmith & Boneham, 2003). The amount of political power, held by individual women, to influence the outcome of the regeneration process is often limited to those with political voices in the community. So, the politics of everyday living impact on individual women in regards to decision made on an institutional level about the place where they live and their community services and resources at the most basic level.

The link between personal and social, as shown above by the many different ways society can impact upon individuals, is complex. Much of the social impact on individuals is made when taking part in everyday activities and constructing lived experience; as health is part of everyday lived experience then social conditions may also impact upon health identity.

Difficulty in understanding social, cultural and political effects may lie in confusion on an individual level. In everyday lived experience, these effects and how they are influencing people are perhaps discreet, thus creating difficulty in expressing this in individual discourse. As Bartky points out:

> The disciplinary power that inscribes femininity is everywhere and it is nowhere; the disciplinarian is everyone yet no one in particular. Women regarded as overweight, for example, report that they are regularly admonished to diet, sometimes by people they scarcely know. (Bartky, 1998, p.74)

There is much feminist literature on these political influences on the way women live and their bodies, and some studies explaining what women say about these politics individually, but few are interactive of the two. This book aims to bring a deconstruction of the personal narrative, the interpersonal relationship and the societal politics of health identity construction sourced from women's accounts of health by asking the question:

*What health considerations have perimenopausal women undergone in lived experience and how have they used these to construct a health identity?*

This question is posed to clarify these considerations and analysis using Murray's levels of personal, interpersonal and institutional analysis, which will bring a deconstructed yet interactive account of what the women in this study feel affects their health. Feminist theory is examined in Chapter 3, and how this impacts on women's lives in the context of living in the world. Additionally, in Chapter 7 the narrative accounts of the women who took part in the study are considered in the context of everyday living in society. This will allow for interpretation of how personal health is affected by critical issues such as inequalities, discrimination, oppression and power dynamics operating in society. The aim is to clarify how these levels show the way health experience is affected and influenced by each of these levels in the same set of narrative accounts, thus identifying a critical agenda in the construction of women's health identity.

## Women's health today – Overview and structure of this book

Even though mainstream health psychology and the associated quantitative testing can be a useful investigation into health, critical health psychology extends the field into the more phenomenological subjective nature of the experience of health and illness and how this interacts with the social nature of health. Whilst the laboratory-based and predetermined questionnaire and survey methods can be used to highlight trends and provide nomothetic demographic data (and are valuable in this context), critical aspects of health psychology enable the investigation of social injustice and inequality, oppression and consequently can inform social change.

By examining the subjective person-centred account of the experience of health and illness, the critical aspects revealed can be applied to health interventions in society. Meaning is an inherent concept of identity and a health identity is constructed by making sense of the meanings of health-related concepts with which we are presented in everyday life. This more subjective methodology will allow this book to reveal an integrated, holistic model of what health and illness is like for the individual, and additionally, through the autobiographical nature of narrative accounts, how this has been built up over time (Greene, 2000).

Essential to critical health psychology, the issue of embodiment becomes pertinent when considering the critical realist position of the intransient nature of the body and the fluid, socially constructed health experience. By studying these personal, interpersonal, and social components together in a holistic manner, critical health psychology goes beyond the objective methodological restraints of mainstream health psychology to provide a theoretical background for the study of complex health, identity and critical issues such as social justice, intervention and social change.

As the aim to investigate the construction of women's health identity, a critical perspective will be taken to look at how societal issues around women's health affect the women who took part in this study. This is to ensure that power dynamics, oppression, and the political and economic context of the women in the study, in addition to investigating any social injustice and inequalities they may have undergone, are considered in addition to the personal narrative account of the woman's health. This will understand better how these issues affect the ways in which women construct their health identity through experience and narrative. The book is divided into three parts, Theory, Voice and Praxis, with Chapter 5 providing a bridge between theory and voice and a model of identity in Chapter 9 forging a bridge between voice and praxis.

## Part I – The Theory

**Chapter 2 – Understanding Women's Health – Health Perspectives:** In this chapter the existing literature regarding women's health is examined. By placing this in the context of the politics of women's bodies, a gap in knowledge regarding a critical, person-centred approach to women's health appears. This can be remedied by the critical approach to women's health supported in the introduction.

**Chapter 3 – Identity Theory and an Interactive Health Identity:** An overview the background of identity theory is explored and a fluid model of identity construction in the light of embodied health experience is proposed in this chapter. Additionally, this chapter will discuss how social theory locates health identity in society.

**Chapter 4 – Feminist as Far as Possible – The Feminist Health Identity and Critical Realism:** Women's social feminist health identity and how women live in the world is considered in this chapter. Feminist standpoint theory is described and used to discuss the material body in terms of health and feminist thinking.

**Chapter 5 – Investigating Women's Health: The Story So Far**: In this chapter, narrative psychology is proposed as a useful tool to critically investigate the health experiences of perimenopausal women. The design of the interview study with women in Oldham is considered and a discussion of qualitative methodology in practice is formed in order to allow the reader to replicate the study or to conduct similar studies.

**Part II – Voice**

**Chapter 6 – Narrative Touchstones of the Storied Perimenopausal Health Identity**: Here the first part of the findings from the interview study are presented. Considering a personal perspective of health, this chapter presents an analysis of perimenopausal women's personal considerations of what health means to them over their whole life and how health is located in their identity.

**Chapter 7 – Reaching Out – Interpersonal Narratives of the Perimenopausal Health Identity**: In this chapter, the second part of the findings from the interview study are analysed. The interpersonal and embodied nature of women's health experience and identity construction in the narrative accounts of the participants is examined for relational differences and commonalities.

**Chapter 8 – Stories of Societal Health – The Impact of Narrated Positional, Situational and Ideological Health Representation**: In this chapter the critical aspects of locating health identity in society are investigated in terms of emerging themes of the politics of lived experience for women.

**Part III – Praxis**

**Chapter 9 – Identity Actions: Bringing about Social Change**: In this chapter different levels of analysis are brought together to reveal a holistic model of identity. This model, which in this book has been applied to women's health identity, is shown to be an overarching model of identity construction which can identify and influence social change.

# Part I

# Theory

The first chapters of this book will deal with theoretical aspects of identity, health and women. The theoretical positions covered in this book cover the disciplines of psychology, sociology, philosophy and biology in order to assess how identity construction can be applied to women's health.

Following discreet chapters covering health psychology, women's health, identity theory and feminist theory a chapter describing how a study was carried out based on this theory highlights methodological issues. A prominent criticism of theory-based work is the absence of a 'real life' context and Chapter 4 acts as a bridge between theory and voice.

# 2
# Understanding Women's Health: Health Perspectives

## What is women's health?

As discussed in the introduction, the concept of health has previously been investigated using traditional positivist methods, based on the biomedical model. Progress made in terms of recognising the psychological and social aspects of health (Engel, 1977) has impacted on the study of health by combining biological, social and psychological effects into investigations, albeit in a fragmented fashion. Whilst this is a useful movement forward, the biopsychosocial model is not gender specific and often based on particular health conditions as an initial point of enquiry.

Women's health involves not just the study of women's biological state or medical conditions. It is important to understand that women's health is an ongoing experience for all women in their everyday lives. Rather than researching the phenomenon of health identity, this project aims to research the experience of health identity and how this is constructed. This involves researching women and interpreting their experiences in the cultural, social and political context in which they take place. Living in the world involves being subject to interactions with other people and taking part in society and this, as discussed in the previous chapter, is all part of women's health. It is important, then, to highlight the individual nature of the health experience for individual women, and consequently the importance of the cultural, social and political aspects of health in society that affect each women individually. This ongoing experience for women is multidimensional and, because of the uniqueness of each individual and the combination of societal aspects that may affect health, it is essential that a starting point of the individual women is taken. Equally essential is that individual health is considered in the context of relationships and society.

Research (Christodoulou, 2006) has found that critical health psychology provides a framework of investigation where understanding the cultural, political and social contexts of health contributes to overarching social change towards wellbeing rather than addressing singular illnesses. This inclusion of health in context enables the study of marginalised groups who often experience more ill health due to oppression and economic disadvantage (Marks et al., 2001). Feminist thinking has identified women as a marginalised and oppressed group. By placing women in this social and cultural context and by critically examining the positioning of women in society in regard to lived experience of health, women's health becomes a pertinent issue for social change.

Therefore, women's health emerges as an important field of study, quite apart from general health. Whilst the reproductive system is often used as a marker for sexual difference in health, women's health in general differs from men's health. Such differences include, on a biological level of analysis, coronary heart disease which involves disease of the heart muscles in both men and women; however pre-menopausal women are protected from heart disease by oestrogen (Luksha & Kublickiene, 2005). In terms of mental health, twice as many women are likely to experience depression than men (Stoppard, 2000). Explaining this difference Stoppard comments that:

> Depression in women is linked to the experience of adversity; especially events and conditions with negative implications for the ongoing quality of women's everyday lives. (Stoppard, 2000, p.407)

In many aspects of society, women are likely to face oppression, and because of the marginalisation of women in society, the social and cultural aspects of women's lived experience are an interactive part of the health experience (Ussher, 2000; Yardley, 1997).

Women's health includes not just material physiological health, but also socially constructed health, particularly in relation to the social construction of gender. In terms of women's health, milestones present in the health lives of all women, such as menstruation, childbirth and menopause provide health constructs that are particular to the experiences of women (Komesaroff, et al., 1997). This integral part of women's health investigates expectation of health and the gendered social roles which help to determine physical and emotional wellbeing (Lees, 2000). Consequently, critical methodology must be employed to evaluate women's health.

## Gendered health: Women's health

In parallel with developments in health psychology and critical health psychology around concepts of power, oppression and social inequality, interest in the field of women's health has increased. Much work has been published on the marginalisation of women's health in the past. Ussher (1991) covers the issue of the objectification of women's bodies and minds in medicine by the imposition of misogynistic social boundaries. Focusing on the discursive practices of construing women's behaviour and the embodiment of this behaviour, Ussher conducts a timeline investigation of how misogynistic practices in society have cast women as 'the other' to the masculine 'norm'. In evaluating 'the feminist critiques' Ussher examines the view that, according to medical data, women '... are more mad than men.' (Ussher, 1991, p.164)

In a critique of the generalisation of statistics, Ussher points out that many of the studies from which data have been gathered were carried out under a patriarchal scientific system and that the specific disorders and gender differences within these are lost in generalisation. Ussher also points out that:

> ... there are virtually as many different theories and arguments in the feminist debate as there are feminists. (Ussher, 1991, p.3)

implying that the positions which women take to explain and reconstruct the medicalisation and objectification of the body through misogyny, are complex. Gender specific health issues, such as pregnancy, the menopause and menstruation (Lyons, 2000) have a history of objectification in mainstream health psychology. Traditionally the woman's body has been portrayed in a negative manner, for example, Freud's concept of the hysterical woman and floating womb (Webster, 1996) and the discourse around the female body has been constructed in order to control by way of subordination.

In their study on meanings of menopause Komesaroff et al. (1997) examined representations of older women in Western society and found that:

> The menopausal woman acquires a variety of social and psychological meanings: she may be 'wise woman', 'oracle', 'priestess' or 'healer'; but she is also 'monster', 'harbinger of man's fate', 'evil force', 'destroyer', 'avenger', 'bitter and twisted hag', 'witch' or 'castrating bitch'. The menopausal women is the personification of the 'abject'. She

> embodies the repressed, unacknowledged, and feared parts of personal identity and societies. (Komesaroff et al., 1997, p.10)

In the objectification of older women in society some aspects of the menopause are perceived negatively by institutionalised power. These in turn are negatively feminised and imposed on older women as a dichotomy to the positive feminisation afforded to younger women by the same power dynamics. Fox Keller (1984) comments that:

> Modern science...is based on a division of emotional and intellectual labour in which objectivity, reason and 'mind' are cast as male and subjectivity, feeling and 'nature' are cast as female! Science involves a radical separation of subject and object and ultimately the domination of mind over nature. The result is a particular conception of science – one that is more suited to men than women. (Fox Keller 1984, p.45)

Following on the theme of 'femaleness' and meaning, Hanson (2001) investigates how the pathologising of aspects of femaleness in biomedical writings is undertaken. Hanson's proposal that:

> ...there is an implicit reliance in biomedicine on the idea that femaleness is pathological hence carcinogenic. (Hanson, 2001, p.469)

was borne out by the findings that, during a comprehensive search of Medline/PubMed, there was:

> ...a greater tendency to see women in sexual terms and to pathologise aspects of femaleness...even extends to more frequent use of the term oestrogen than testosterone in exclusively male cancer sites. (Hanson, 2001, p.471).

This illustrates the ongoing objectification of women's health through the highlighting of sex difference. These stereotypical ideals of a binary opposite gender division is in dispute in poststructural terms, as the postmodern model of gender is not fixed stereotypically in so far as no two people have a unique identity. Therefore, no two people have an identically constructed gender identity, suggesting multiple gender identities.

It has been suggested that gender is in fact heavily influenced by external cultural stereotypes and expectations in experiential terms

(Courtenay, 2000). As health is highly gendered, due to gender difference in experience of health, it can be proposed that socially constructed health identity is vulnerable to the same gender stereotypes and expectations (Sixsmith & Boneham, 2003). This is evident in studies of men's health by Courtney (2000) which suggests that in order to maintain a macho stereotype; men will not seek health advice or curb risk-taking behaviour if the consequences are seen to be on a feminine behaviour trajectory. The health-related results of this construction of masculinity are illustrated by the mortality rates and causes in studies of men's health. Similarly, in a paper by Lee and Owens (2002) the focus is on both the individual and social aspects of gendered men's health. The paper argues that risk taking in men is generally seen in society, particularly in law pertaining to criminal behaviour, as freely chosen behaviour and that there is:

> ...little awareness of the role of social constructions in men's choices. (Lee & Owens, 2002, p.209)

According to literature on men's health, the risk-taking stereotype of macho behaviour does in fact have an influence on men's health-related behaviour.

Conversely, the construction of femininity from representations in society and culture promote the discourse of care and nurture through the use of binary opposite representations (Bonner et al., 1992). These represent women as the opposite of the macho stereotype, and as the 'other' caregiver to men's dominant political and economic roles in society. Rudman and Glick (2001) examine gender stereotyping and the backlash towards agentic (e.g. self-directed or independent as opposed to those reliant or dependant on others) women in their paper discussing discrimination in the workplace. The authors find that agentic women are penalised in the workplace due to the perception of a female stereotype of 'niceness'.

However, women's health studies have shown that although the care and nurture stereotype influences women's perception of their role, women do in fact take part in risky health-related behaviour. Critical health psychologists recognise that whilst there are gender differences in stress-related behaviour and risk taking, studies regarding substance abuse, smoking, heart disease and eating disorders are inclusive of women. Such studies have shown the physiological effects of risk-taking behaviour such as smoking, alcohol consumption and eating disorders (see Hardy et al., 1999, 2000). Even so, it is difficult to dig deeper into the identity to see why, if women's identities are constructed in the direction of nurture and care and therefore invested healthy behaviour, that, in so many cases, many women are living unhealthy lives. Consequently, recent investigations into women's health have sought to find meaning and discourse behind health-related behaviour.

Women's health is more than a stereotypical objectification of the body and gender pathology; women's health takes in all the aspects of women's socially constructed health identity: biopsychosocial aspects of health, relationships, interactions within society, socio-political struggles and the considerations of the disadvantages and, less illustrated advantages of the ageing, healthy woman in society. Taking these factors into account, the study of women's health would be furthered in terms of understanding by development of critical methodology employing an integrated approach to investigate what contributes to the construction of woman's health identity, throughout her life. Investigation into lived experience of women and how their health identity is expressed through not solely the magnification of the medical discourse, but also the effects of other important discourses present in society, such as family and feminist discourse, would elucidate the holistic lived health experience of women. In particular, the way that women's bodies are politicised in the health arena, and women's response to this, allow examination of the interaction between the personal and the social. Investigation into this would provide a critical framework that illuminates and clarifies the project of critical health psychology by highlighting the marginalisation of women by oppression, social inequality and power dynamics present in lived health experiences of women.

By pointing the focus of the medical model to areas where it would be better applied, and by allowing the voices of women to narrate the whole life narrative of health, a balanced interpretation of health identity construction could emerge from the subjective standpoint of health identity as opposed to the patient. Despite this, as can be seen above from recent literature, much of the study of women's health remains based in the biological and biopsychosocial models of health psychology, ignoring the integrated cultural, political and social aspects of women's lived health experiences.

## Non-reproductive health in women

Women experience general health problems outside of the context of reproductive health (Ussher, 2000). These non-reproductive health problems such as heart disease, diabetes, smoking, alcohol and drug use, cancer and digestive disease are often generalised and studied from an illness-based perspective in the biological model of health which focuses on the material body. This does not take into account sex differences or gender constructions and their effects on the general health of women. Because most of the problems are physiological and are the remit of medicine in order to cure a disease, a scientific approach is often used to investigate their impact.

More recent developments have shown that non-reproductive illness in women's health is markedly different to the same general illness in men's health due to biological differences. For example, Dhiman and Chawlw (2006) studied the effects of oestrogen on gall bladder disease in women. This study was quantitative in design and investigated the effects of female sex hormones on cholelithiasis, a disease of the gall bladder that is more common in women than in men. The findings indicate that naturally produced oestrogen, such as that produced in pregnancy, contributes to the higher incidence of this disease in women. Additionally, the hormone replacement therapy that includes oestrogen promotes this disease in post-menopausal women. This shows that fluctuating oestrogen in women's bodies make the incidence of gall bladder disease in women higher than in men because of sex differences.

As discussed earlier construction of meaning and health around women's bodies are subject to power dynamics in society and these politics are highly relevant to gendered health. This suggests that whilst non-reproductive health in women is not gendered in medical terms, some sex differences related to the physiological reproductive system exist and affect health. Additionally, the complex differences in lived experience between women as suggested by Lawlor et al. (2004), and indeed between men and women, suggest that sex differences and gender divide general health.

## Mental health and women

Women's mental health is an issue that has been widely researched in terms of individual women and predefined medical conditions (Stoppard, 2000). For example, Oedegaard et al. (2006) investigated the association of depression and anxiety with migraines and comment that women are more often affected by all three of these experiences than men. In this survey-based study, the authors suggest that women are more affected because of differences in sex hormones between women and men. However, no societal or cultural considerations were included in the design of this study, implying that issues of sex difference were prioritised over gender differences.

Researchers have recognised that by taking a critical feminist approach to research into mental health, women's experiences and socially, politically and culturally situated health provide an understanding of the impact of mental health issues on women's lives. For example, issues of abortion are heavily grounded in social and political societal discourses as Fergusson et al. (2006) have shown. They investigated the incidence of mental health issues in young women (ages 15–25) who had had an abortion. This study considered the history of pregnancy and abortion amongst the sample and experiences such as suicidal behaviour, depression, anxiety and substance abuse, over the study period.

In line with the biopsychosocial model of health, the study also examined 'childhood, family and related confounding factors' (p.16). This complex statistical study using a sample of 520 young women found that there is an association of increased risks of 'mental health problems' following abortion in young women. However, Denious and Russo (2000) remind us that:

> It is important to remember that the meaning of abortion is socially constructed. This common experience in women's lives can be made to seem wrong and shameful, and women in turn can suffer from this social construction. (Denious & Russo, 2000, p.437)

In remembering that the meaning of abortion is socially constructed, it is important to be mindful that the meaning of mental health and how it is pathologised is also socially constructed. By taking a critical stance, the way mental health is pathologised is not a personal position of the author of this book; rather this pathological construction lies with the authors of the papers cited. Their pathological construction of mental health has been highlighted here so as to point out their construction of the inevitable pathology of medicalised mental health.

Russo and Denious (1998) studied the incidence of 'mental health problems' following abortion, and, using a critical design to qualitatively investigate this, they found that the abortion experience itself has no significant association with mental health. Taking a feminist standpoint and including the influence of abortion politics in the research agenda would extend Fergusson et al.'s (2006) biopsychosocial investigation towards a critical evaluation inclusive of the social, political and cultural factors. This critical approach elucidates the lived experience of abortion in context, to expose strong agendas of the oppression of women regarding reproductive rights and attitudes to abortion in society which may influence any decisions made. This valuable insight into the experience of abortion is a conscious raising matter that critical health psychologists could use to inform social change and meaning making discourse about social justice and women's choice and freedom.

An observation of these investigations is that even though Denious and Russo published their observations in 2000 and clearly extended health psychology in this area to include a critical approach, use of the biopsychosocial model to investigate mental health issues associated with abortion persists within Fergusson et al.'s 2006 study. This perhaps indicates a resistance to explore the oppression of women in a political sense because of the power of the positivist model that underpins the medical model. This confirms the patriarchal nature of the medical model and biopsychosocial model of health psychology.

Women's non-reproductive health and mental health continue to be generalised over sex differences in symptomisation. Consequently, slow progress has been made in these areas in moving towards a position where women's health is considered an exclusive field of study. Women's reproductive health is clearly marked by sex differences, and scientific study of these areas highlight female reproductive physiology, particularly hormonal influences associated with menstruation, pregnancy, childbirth and menopause as underlying health problems (Ussher, 2000). In the following section, the literature and methodology found to be concerned with these milestones of women's health are reviewed. In particular, the menopause and perimenopause are examined as this is a central concern of women and their identity, and methodologies associated with the study of women's reproductive health.

## Reproductive health – Periods, pregnancy and childbirth

Reproductive health milestones begin with periods and the menstrual cycle. As women progress through puberty and periods start, the reproductive cycle becomes an issue for health. Roberts (2000) comments that:

> In everyday experience in the West, women put a range of negative experiences down to sex hormones. Hormones are used to explain the edginess of PMT. (Roberts, 2000, p.283)

The focus on reproductive health issues presents a difficult dilemma for feminist thinking when critically investigating women's reproductive health. Whilst it is clear that hormones are part of sex differences, they do not solely create them, nor do they account for gender differences between men and women (Roberts, 2000). In addition to this, the influence of culture and society's impact on the construction of pre-menstrual syndrome (PMS) which is also medicalised as pre-menstrual tension (PMT), and in turn how it is experienced personally, is substantial. It is therefore important to evaluate both personal and social aspects of PMS.

Research indicates that much of the research into women's reproductive health, the influence of the medical model of health's focus on physiological bodies has granted sex hormones excessive potency for determining reproductive health issues (Harraway, 1991). For example, Misri and Kendrick (2006) studied the use of the paroxatine, an anti-depressant drug, for the treatment of pre-menstrual dysphoric disorder. The authors describe this severe form of PMS as occurring during the luteal phase of the menstrual cycle which is associated with a fall in oestrogen. Whilst commenting that the symptoms may include depressed mood, irritability, and anxiety, recommendations for the use of selective serotonin reuptake inhibitors (SSRI'S) and in particular paroxetine are made. This study completely excludes any social, cultural, or political aspects of not just social constructions of pre-menstrual dysphoric disorder, but also depression, anxiety and irritability which negates lived experience of pre-menstrual women and focuses solely on biological factor and consequent treatment with drugs. Because of this focus on the medical model of health, socio-cultural understandings of PMS are under-researched. Reilly (2000) considers biopsychosocial research into PMS.

Reilly discusses the construction of PMS as a psychiatric or medical problem and concludes that if research is to critically understand PMS then qualitative investigations must take place. This is to deconstruct the societal, cultural and political meanings of PMS, understand how these have been imposed on women, and understand how women experience PMS in terms of these. Swann and Ussher (1995) support the acknowledgement of PMS as a gendered problem and suggest that more attention should be paid to the relationship between PMS and identity. Additionally, the political nature of PMS construction in society around women's capability to work and interact in relationships must be investigated alongside this. In these terms, Martin (2006) comments on the medicalisation of PMS and how it is perceived in society.

Further to this, when the social, cultural and political issues around PMS are better understood a physiological examination of PMS outside the medicalised problematic meanings of menstruation and PMS would help to understand the biological process experienced by women. However, to date, and as shown by Misri and Kendrick's (2006) study above, many published investigations into PMS are still dominated by the medical model of health.

Pregnancy is another aspect of women's health that has become medicalised. Gross (2000) comments that:

> The pathologisation of female functioning in pregnancy is relayed in the equation of pregnancy with sickness, in employment legislation, for example. (Gross, 2000, p.297)

Gross discusses the passive role of pregnant women as they attend antenatal clinics and during the labour period, where women are often attached to medical machines that monitor the progress of the labour. In addition to this, the dualist medical model is reinforced in the metaphor of the woman's body as a vessel for the baby, and the responsibility imposed on the body as a healthy vessel as a predictor of the fitness of the baby at birth. Even though this monitoring of health is necessary during pregnancy for optimum wellbeing, it adds to the social construction of pregnancy as a problematic event (Gross, 2000). Because of the medical nature of health monitoring at antenatal classes and deliveries in hospitals, pregnancy remains entrenched in the medical model of health, and recent published investigations support this. For example, Cuevas and Sanz (2006) investigated the safety of SSRI's in pregnancy and comment that:

> ...depression has a high prevalence in pregnant women (around 10%) and approximately one-half of the pregnancies are unplanned, making necessary that physicians have to know the risks associated with the decision to use this kind of antidepressant during pregnancy. (Cuevas & Sanz, 2006, p.18)

Their study, which examines the effects of serotonin transmission on embryo development, is undoubtedly useful when SSRI's are used in pregnancy. A more pertinent critical analysis of depression in pregnancy would aim to understand why around 10 per cent of pregnant women are depressed, if this is solely due to pregnancy (as implied in the investigation above) and what contributes to this depression.

The studies above have illustrated that many aspects of women's health are at best investigated from a biopsychosocial perspective and that there is limited movement towards a critical evaluation of women's health, which includes social, cultural, and political constructions that impact on lived experience. The generalised medical aspects of women's general and mental health and women's health in terms of reproductive health all contribute to a lifelong journey through health during which time a personal perspective of health is cumulatively formed. This health identity, which is further investigated in Chapter 3, is well formed by the onset of the menopause, and the aim of this book is to investigate how the stages or milestones of women's health have impacted on a health identity. As the women in this study are perimenopausal, that is, around the time of the menopause, in the following section progress made in study of the menopause and the perimenopause is reviewed in detail.

## Reproductive health – The menopause and the perimenopause

In order to expose the construction of a health identity, the women in the interviews included in this book are perimenopausal and have a mature lived health experience in terms of chronological time. As a health-related milestone which occurs relatively late in life and to which women look as a watershed in their health life, the perimenopause, or the time around the menopause, is a gateway to an insight into how women, up to this point, have collected health experiences and applied them in their whole lives to construct a health identity.

The study of the menopause as a health milestone in women's life has run in parallel with developments in health psychology. Because of the gendered nature of health and, as explained above, the objectification of women's bodies through patriarchal practices in biomedicine, the experience of menopause became similarly medicalised.

Rostosky and Travis (1996) comment on the subject of the dominance of the biomedical model in menopause research. A literature search of online publications between 1984 and 1994 found that a large proportion of the papers and articles described menopause in a negative context. Concepts highlighted by this study were: menopausal women as 'the opposite sex', 'the sicker sex' and 'the weaker sex'. The authors argue on the basis of this that:

> ...the emphasis on biological explanations of women and women's life experiences lead to negative stereotypes about women. (Rostosky & Travis, 1996, p.301)

and that menopause is often viewed as a problem due to these negative constructions.

Gannon and Stevens (1998) examined the mass media for the development of media attitudes towards the menopause from 1981 to 1994 and found that, although there had been an increase in articles relating to the menopause, it was a subject of relatively minor media interest. Also, the findings indicated that there was a focus on the negative aspects of the menopause, in line with Rostosky and Travis' (1996) research. In addition to this, Gannon and Stevens highlight the increasing interest in hormone replacement therapy (HRT). HRT has been developed as a 'cure' for menopausal symptoms over the past two decades and the authors have noted that:

> Research designed to investigate the menopause as a medical disease in the context of patriarchal ideology is consistent with the prevailing ideology of government and industry and is, therefore, likely to be funded; the subsequent research is, first, published in journals that rely on pharmaceutical advertising, and, second 'packaged' for easy use by the media. (Rostosky & Travis, 1996, p.307)

The implications of this for health psychology are that the biomedical model of the menopause may be artificially sustained by the prescription of HRT as an elixir for media produced stereotypical negative aspects of the menopause.

Pharmaceutical advertisements, however, have, according to Kaufert and Lock (1997) made some effort to change the 1970s advertisements for HRT and other menopausal remedies of the 'depressed and sickly looking woman' into a '1990's version of the menopausal woman shown as glowing with fitness' (Kaufert & Lock, 1997, p.80). Kaufert and Lock look at how the menopausal woman is represented in these images in order to highlight the balance between the medical model and the associated economic and political power of pharmaceutical companies, and the effect on the ageing population of women. The findings of this report are as follows:

> The medical model of what happens to the menopausal woman is not to be confused with the reality of women's experience and yet the two are intimately intertwined. How physicians and others think about the menopause and treat the menopausal women depends on whatever is the currently accepted model of the menopausal woman. This model also determines how menopausal women see themselves and how they are expected to look and behave. (Kaufert & Lock, 1997, p.83)

So, in common with the main aspects of mainstream health psychology, earlier models of the menopause have constructed the menopause in a biomedical, negative context with a comprehensive symptom list and as a disease of the body. Accordingly, as health psychology has moved on to the biopsychosocial model, the notion that it has been recognised that women's menopausal experience is not limited to the cessation of menses is worth investigation. Although the biomedical aspects of the menopause are real and cannot be ignored, socio-cultural implications of women's lived experiences must somehow be integrated into the biomedical menopausal model.

Diverting slightly from the examination of the biomedical model of menopause, at this point the anthropological angle of investigations into the menopause are considered as this highlights cultural differences in menopausal concepts. Lock (1998) conducted a comparative study of menopause in women from Japan and from North America and Europe. As well as acknowledging the end of menstruation as the medical signifier of the menopause, Lock explains that the accompanying biological and socio-cultural changes associated with menopause are not universal. Lock's study, using questionnaires, interviews and focus groups, found that in Japan there is no specific word for the Western biomedical model of menopause as an event centred around the cessation of menses. Rather, the Japanese word 'konenki' describes a transitional time in terms of lived experience around the menopause. Further, the standardised symptom list of the western biomedical model of the menopause, invariably including 'hot flushes/flashes' varied considerably from the symptoms reported by the Japanese women. Additionally, there is no Japanese word for 'hot flash/flush' that signifies the rarity of this Western symptom in Japanese menopausal women. Lock fields the counter argument often used to dismiss these culturally constructed differences, that of the recent advent of the menopause because women are living longer aided by technological interventions, by arguing that high mortality rates have confounded life expectancy figures, and evidence has shown that archaeologists have discovered remains of old women since prehistoric nomadic societies.

This supports further the concept that biology is not the sole signifier of menopause and that in fact menopause is more accurately viewed as a complex biopsychosocio-cultural process. As a consequence of the acceptance of a more integrated model of menopause, and in line with the development of the biopsychosocial model in health psychology, investigations have been carried out and published into more qualitative aspects of the menopause.

To bring menopausal research in line with the biopsychosocial model in health psychology, Bowles (1990) proposed a model of menopause which involved evaluation of current cultural representation of menopause to identify how these representations affect women's expectations regarding ageing and mid life. Beliefs, values and assumptions about women at midlife are the basis of Bowles' model and this is a major development in acknowledging the experiential aspects of the menopause as opposed to simply the physiologically given symptoms.

Research on the menopause has continued in line with Bowles thinking and has advanced the model. This research is mainly concerned with the comparison of the biomedical model of menopause and the paradigm of menopause as a natural developmental process that signals a life transition (Gannon & Ekstrom, 1993).

Gannon and Ekstrom (1993) argue that attitudes towards the menopause are dependant on the model of menopause available to women. As previously stated, the biomedical model of the menopause as 'diseased' creates a negative attitude. However, citing Bowles' model (1990) of menopausal attitudes, the authors have investigated, through questionnaires, how attitudes towards the menopause change over time. They found that younger women whose sole experience of the menopause was the media and biomedical representations of health had mostly negative attitudes towards the menopause, whereas older women who had their own experience of menopause to draw on were generally more positive in attitude towards the menopause. The authors conclude that:

> Women, menopausal or not, will benefit more from controlling their own fertility, pregnancies and menopause than from having their bodies and psyches 'guided' by 'experts'. (Gannon and Ekstrom, 1993, p.286)

This observation leads on to a dilemma facing researchers wishing to further study the menopause in terms of a more integrated model and from a more woman-centred perspective. Health psychology has made a linear development towards a more holistic way of integrating the experiential aspects of health with biomedical considerations. However, with the advent of HRT, the biomedical model of the menopause has been brought back to the fore, with HRT being cited as a 'cure-all' for any symptoms the menopause may bring and also other future health considerations such as osteoporosis and heart disease. This is an example of political and cultural aspects of the power dynamics of construction of women's health. Barbre (1998) comments that:

> ...menopause does not occur in a vacuum. It, like other events resulting form women's reproductive biology, menstruation and childbirth,

> for instance, is given meaning and value by the culture within which it occurs. (Barbre, 1998, p.243)

Barbre suggests that the promotion of HRT treatment is a response to society's objectification of women and that HRT helps to perpetuate the overtly feminine construction of women in Western Society. The UK government has been keen to promote HRT and has commissioned a number of reports into women's health at midlife.

Jubilee Women was a project from the Societal Issues Research Centre (2001) in conjunction with 'HRT Aware' and investigated 'fiftysomething' women. The aim of this research was to investigate how women felt that HRT benefited them and their experience of the menopause. The study used mixed methods and the published report includes interviews with celebrities and a female GP who had taken HRT. The findings of the report emphasise the benefits of HRT and even claim that the research has revealed a new 'elite' – nicknamed the HRHs (Hormone-Rich and Happy). According to this research, the menopause can be a positive and uplifting experience, particularly with the help of HRT. A major critique of this report is the focus on the benefits of HRT without a balanced investigation into the risks of HRT.

This economic and political interest in women's health is typical of patriarchal and misogynistic attempts to medicalise and control women's lives. By promoting HRT as a cure for the menopause and other related health problems, agencies may be encouraging women further into the external control of the medical world by creating a reliance on prescribed drugs. As the promotion of menopause as a life transition is not in the interests of biomedical patriarchy it is difficult to secure research funding into menopausal issues which do not involve aspects of biomedical and HRT promotion. Additionally, the NHS will, in future years, struggle to cope with the growing demands on resources if HRT continues to be perceived as a biological solution to menopausal women's health problems and this would relieve the requirement to focus on other more qualitative aspects of women's health.

Also, HRT is not without its risks. In addition to the proposed benefits to health and relief of menopausal symptoms, there is an increased risk of breast and ovarian cancer associated with the use of HRT. In 2002 a longitudinal study in progress in the USA, conducted by the Women's Health Initiative (2002) into the effects of HRT, was halted due to preliminary negative findings. As a consequence it is clear that women have serious decisions to make about the pros and cons of taking HRT to make before they make a final decision over whether to take it or not. It is clear from this discussion that both individual, personal decision-making and socio-political influences in society concerning women and their health affect the prevailing position in HRT. Taking into account the power dynamics in operation in society through agencies and NHS promotion of HRT and the risks involved, the question of information available for individual decision-making arises.

Stephens et al. (2002) consider the discursive construction of HRT and acknowledge that:

> The use of hormone replacement therapy involves complex decisions for mid-aged women owing to controversy about the meaning of the menopause and uncertainty regarding risks and benefits. (Stephens et al., 2002, p.347)

This study highlights that HRT within discourses of the menopause has become a socially constructed medium by which women make decisions and judgements about the biomedical model of the menopause.

In a study concerning menopausal healthcare interventions, Clinkinbeard et al. (1999) state that women often employ other strategies for dealing with menopausal symptoms and general healthcare in mid life. These include taking vitamins, exercise, herbal remedies and food supplements. In an open-ended question included in the questionnaire, women stated that they 'wanted better knowledge of HRT' and asked 'when their periods would end with HRT'. The conclusions of the study, which appeared to be in favour of HRT intervention, recommended that women should be better informed about managing their health in conjunction with the medical world.

Whilst menopausal research and models of menopause are firmly entrenched in the biomedical paradigm promulgated by promotion of HRT, advances in methodology have been made in line with critical thinking in health psychology to focus on more qualitative methods.

In one influential study, Griffiths (1999) used thematic analysis to analyse women's control and choice regarding use of HRT. This investigation was more women-centred, using interviews and focus groups and, more importantly, analysing the data from the viewpoint of:

> The menopause being limited to the action of the women and by changes in society. (Griffiths, 1999, p.470)

The results show that many of the women in the study resisted medicalisation of the menopause, preferring to take medication as a last resort.

A possible implication of this for study of the menopause is that research, which is designed to measure the medicalised menopause, may exclude the actual lived experience of menopausal women. By focusing on quantity-based methodology and using pre-determined questions concerning HRT, cause and effect of symptoms and ignoring the effects of any cumulative health identity, subjectivity may be minimised.

As shown by exploring the literature on menopause, the parallels with the developments in health psychology and the development of critical health psychology are not mirrored entirely. The medicalisation of the menopause, confounded by the patriarchal control of women's health as a negatively gendered concept, continues to hold back research into this important area of health identity. Lived experience and the inevitable progress through the women's reproductive health milestones, general health and mental health are a cumulative experience. Reproductive milestones such as menstruation, childbirth and menopause punctuate women's lived health experience both physiologically through the material body and psychologically through the meaning ascribed to these through discourse. These milestones are therefore part of 'what it is to be a woman' in terms of health, and can be seen as part of the meaning of the self in identity. This suggests that women's health identity may be a cumulative experience comprising both material aspects of health and socially constructed experiences of health. Therefore, the study of a singular element of experience would be better critically evaluated in terms of past experiences of health and health in the context of social, cultural and political representation in society. The construction of the menopause as a singular occurrence signified by the biological sign of the cessation of menses has moved on into investigations into more women-centred studies of the whole of the climacteric based on women's health milestones discussed in this chapter.

Conversely, literature shows that HRT issues continue to place the menopause in the biomedical model of medical control. In very recent developments, the term perimenopause has become a more useful description of the subjective elements combined with the physiological elements of the menopause.

## The perimenopause

The perimenopause is a term used to describe the time around the menopause. Research describes this time as a period from around 35 years of age to 55 years of age when hormone imbalance causes disruption to the menstrual cycle and certain typical symptoms are experienced such as irregular periods, hot flushes and anxiety (Burger et al., 2002; Hudson, 2002; Samisoe, 2002).

Acknowledgement in health psychology is that menopause as more than a single biomedical event has led to the elongation of the period leading up to the cessation of the menses and consequently, consideration of women's symptoms and experiences of this time have been studied. The difference between the menopause and the perimenopause, however, lies within the medicalisation of the menopause in material terms and the socially constructed nature of the perimenopause in temporal and experiential terms. Where the meaning of the menopause is still grounded heavily in biology, the perimenopause is based on the transitional 'time around the menopause' which encompasses the biological menopause itself with the ending of the menses and medicalised symptomology along with an experience of how the menopause affects women over a period of time. This presents an opportunity for thinking around women's health to extend menopause study into the realm of critical health psychology by attempting to understand the social construction of menopause in society without losing the biologically realist aspect of the menopause.

However, the vast majority of these studies have been conducted within the biomedical model of cause and effect of physiological symptoms (Rostosky & Travis, 1996). Many concern contraception and HRT, in addition to other mid-life illnesses, and menopause and perimenopause are mentioned only as a passing acknowledgement of the chronological ages of the sample. This suggests that the perimenopause is still firmly grounded in, at best, the biopsychosocial model of health psychology.

Published journal papers concern the concept of the perimenopause as a transitional time around the menopause or take a qualitative stance on the experiences of women around this time. Many of these papers are concerned with HRT and physical symptoms as an extension of the menopause in a quantitative cause and effect way, rather than considering the feelings and emotional concerns of women passing through a developmental phase supported by the low trend in use of the term perimenopause as mentioned above. The literature is also lacking a feminist perspective of the menopause, which suggests that a critical approach to the menopause is not included, ignoring any issues of social oppression and/or power dynamics underpinning women's health. In addition to this, family history and communication of health ideas is not taken into consideration in most of the literature.

In common with general menopause studies on the tone of menopausal self help literature (Lyons & Griffin, 2002), much of the literature available through general internet search engines is biomedical and negative in nature, often offering commercial 'cures' for menopausal symptoms.

## Understanding women's health – Women doing health

Developments in health psychology, gendered health and the perimenopause suggests that during the past two decades tremendous advances towards a more integrated model of critical health psychology has been made. However, any critical agenda must include participation in health and the voices of the women experiencing gendered health in terms of both reproductive health and general health which are not represented in theory. Lived health experience of women includes 'doing' health on a daily basis, in the context of Mark et al.'s, (2001) 'health as a state of being' (p.4) and in the context of relating their health status to themselves and to others (Frank, 2000b). This constant daily, lived account of health status is the autobiographical narrative (Frank, 2000a) that stories 'what health means', and the identity of health in the unique individual account (McAdams, 1993). The manner in which women construct their health identity from this person-centred perspective (Rogers, 1951) and the impact of representations of health in society on health identity are consequently frequently absent from advancing theories of women's health despite recommendations by critical health theorist for their inclusion. This brings us back to the central question of the book which aims to address this issue by asking:

*What health considerations have perimenopausal women undergone in lived experience and how have they used these to construct a health identity?*

This book will use a critical approach to health. Social, cultural and political representations of health will be investigated through the women's accounts of lived experience and will empower women, whose voices usually go unheard in society because of the disempowering effect of living in a deprived social and economic community, to take part in a project where their experiences are important and valued. Because investigation of lived experience presents opportunities to investigate health critically, and much of the previous research into women's health, as discussed above, has focused on the medical and biopsychosocial models of health psychology, a new approach is needed.

Murray and Campbell (2003), in discussing a new approach for health psychology, call for:

> ...critical practice at different levels of intervention. They distinguish between individual, group and organisational and community and societal levels of analysis and intervention. (Murray & Campbell, 2003, p.231)

This suggests that a new approach must be found to investigate health in a critical way. This should combine levels of lived experience that impact on health, that is, personal, interpersonal and social levels. This presents a research dilemma because, as discussed in the previous two chapters, health is best investigated in a way that recognises its unique and personal nature but also recognises that there are commonalities in health experiences that affect us all. The biological and biopsychosocial models of health have so far not included an investigation of the personal nature of health. As previously discussed, both are entrenched in the medical model of health and tend to generalise about health. Mostly using predefined categories of health (such as stress and pathologically constructed mental health), these models do not progress far from the cause and effect model of health. It is clear, however, that even though narrow and shallow variables may be used, often there are commonalities of health found and in context, these can be used to understand health issues that many people may have in common.

Conversely, taking a personal and unique approach to health would mean that each person's health would be entirely different to the next person. As this is clearly not the case, it would be more productive to start with a person-centred (Rogers, 1951) approach to health and, after analysis of several people's holistic health experiences, try to find any health commonalities that relate to personal, interpersonal and social aspects of health. This way any common health issues identified would be emergent from the personal and unique experiences of the people who were interviewed. This would provide a way to address Murray's contention of a critical investigation, as it would take as a starting point of lived experience and provide and understanding of what holistic health means when living in society with other people. This would incorporate a political and social context of health.

Whilst this way of investigating health is not generalisable in the way results arise from the biological and biopsychosocial models, the work described in this book aims to understand what the women involved are experiencing in the context of a disadvantaged community. By investigating these experiences that emerge from the accounts in terms of themes, tones and images it will be possible to interpret and understand how they are linked to personal, interpersonal and social issues of health and how these contribute to the construction of a health identity. Murray and Campbell also state that:

> Much work remains to be done in developing *actionable* understandings of the complex individual-society dialectic underlying social equalities. (Murray & Campbell, 2003, p.235)

In this work, which takes place in a deprived and disadvantaged social and economic area of Oldham in the North West of England, Murray's 'social equalities' may well be translated into social inequalities for the women taking part, in addition to gender constructed power dynamics. In order to investigate these issues, a deconstruction of health experiences of perimenopausal women in terms of analysis of the holistic life construction of health identity takes place. This is in order to assess what considerations women in this study take into account to construct and reconstruct their holistic health identity through the personal, interpersonal, ideological and positioned levels of analysis of health experience (Murray, 2000). As a starting point, the next chapter examines how identity is constructed, how identity is positioned in society and what this means for women's health identity.

# 3
# Identity Theory and an Interactive Health Identity

## Introduction

In order to understand women's health identity, how identity is formed must be investigated so as to understand the process. In the following chapter, identity formation and methodology employed in the investigation of identity formation will be considered. The concept that personal models of identity and social models of identity are insufficient to separately explain identity construction in the light of a critical approach will be discussed, and a model of identity which includes both social and personal aspects of health identity will be proposed as a more appropriate approach to investigate identity construction. In the following sections, identity will be introduced and compared with personal and social models of identity to arrive at an interactive health identity that includes the location of identity within society through investigation of social theory.

## What is identity?

Identity is a complex concept in psychology and the literature concerning identity is comprehensive and varied in nature. Before considering different models, it is important to establish that identity is a personal entity that applies to all individuals. It is also something which is located in the social world and embodied in relationships with others (Woodward, 2004). Identity is a concept that answers the question 'who am I' by 'who I am' in everyday talk, thought and behaviour and affects all parts of everyday life. By linking the personal self to the social world, identity connects the uniqueness of personal experience to the ordered social world. Because of this connection, identity is not formed purely by personal choice to identify with certain aspects of everyday life, but is also influenced by societal representations that are outside our control. An example of this is decision-making around HRT discussed in the previous chapter. Whilst people feel that they are choosing the kinds of identities they take up, they are also being shaped by possibilities (or lack of possibilities) in the world in which they live. In this sense, identity is the combination of what I would want for myself and how I see myself, how others see me and how this is possible in the context of available opportunities in my world (Woodward, 2004). This holistic proposal for identity is linked to a critical psychological approach, as the impact of societal possibilities and opportunities plays a large part in the shaping of identity and the consideration of this is important in investigating how people construct their identities. As identity is a concept that is personal but also shaped by the social world, a starting point for the study of identity can be the description of identity awareness by the experiencing person.

Therefore, the study of identity is concerned with conscious awareness of the world and attention to what is involved in 'being a person' (Harre, 1983). Identity theory and its concern with personal lived experience have historically been investigated from two main perspectives: the self as embodied in the social world and the individual self. More recent thinking aims to provide an explanation of identity as a seamless process constantly acting between the self and the social world, providing a more holistic model in conjunction with social theory. In the following chapter, these models of identity will be explored in relation to health identity.

## How is identity formed?

Identity construction occurs through interaction with the social world (Woodward, 2004). People are aware to one degree or another that they are living in the world and that the world impacts them. They then act on the world accordingly. Which part of the world they internalise, and which part of that internalised knowledge they embody in the world as a consequence constitutes the process of identity formation (Burkitt, 1998). This has been studied in several different ways and identity theory is concerned with the processes by which identity is formed.

Identity from the personal perspective asks the question, 'who am I?' and Western thought separates and fences in this question marking the individual as separate from society (Burkitt, 1998). Research, therefore, into personal identity, may take the individual as the basis of enquiry. Identity study involving personal aspects of the self focuses on the question of 'who am I?' from a perspective of who I feel I am, in personal terms. This excludes the considerations of social, cultural and political societal locations of identity. Conversely, society is important in identity study as individual identities impact on society, asking the question 'what is the world?' just as society impacts personal identity. Research into society, therefore, may involve study of identity as embodied in the world. The focus on societal impacts on identity, however, excludes the personal and unique nature identity of identity formation and construction.

In the following sections personal and social models of the self will be explored and, in order to take a critical approach to identity, how these two aspects of self must interact to form a fluid model of identity. In addition to this, social theory and the ways that identity can be located in society is included to form a link to lived experience.

Mead (1934) makes a useful comment on the internal self as a starting point by focusing on the processes that are involved in linking the internal and external selves. Mead suggests that identities are created in a social context through 'the looking-glass self'. This consists of the 'I' the inner self and the 'me' as the self in the social world. The 'I' perception of self-identity is a fluid process of constantly reflecting from the external world of 'me' and how the social world imposes aspects of identity onto 'me'. This model of fluid, ever-reflective identity is important as it renders both biological/behavioural and the social construction explanations as partial. Therefore, a suitable methodological approach, which takes the personal perspective as the starting point and takes both the social and the personal construction of the self and clarifies the embodiment of identity in the world, must be used in order to fully study identity construction. This personal starting point is necessary as identity is unique and personal. In addition to this personal starting point, the location of identity in society and their interaction is of equal importance in constructing health identity for perimenopausal women.

## Personal perspectives of the self

The qualitative study of identity has been widely developed in the past two decades. Taking the personal account as a starting point, it is possible to look for meaning, emotions and attitudes; these give insight into how sense is made of the world and how this is internalised into the identity. However, with this ontological switch to the self as subject, concepts of the self become important.

### Phenomenology and experiential psychology

Phenomenology provides a method of investigating identity from an experiential standpoint (May, 1983). According to the phenomenological perspective, it is possible to introspect and identify feelings experienced as a person, and of awareness of the social world. As conscious awareness is not quantifiable, but reliant on each person's own interpretation of their inner thoughts, introspection and the expression of the results of this introspection are considered to be the 'data' available for study in this experiential perspective.

As phenomenology and experiential psychology are grounded in consciousness, awareness, intentionality and thought process, they are inevitably linked to philosophy. William James described awareness of experience as 'the stream of consciousness' (James, 1890, in 1950 reprint). James suggested that consciousness consists of different levels of experience and has a continually changing quality. The implications for identity in James' experiential theory are that our personal experiences built over time and, through knowledge generation of these experiences and feelings, we are able to live as an agent in the world. The social world is accounted for by explaining the objective and the subjective as co-constructed and the concept of intentionality, where experience is constituted by directing and owning subjective consciousness and perception towards objects when creating meaning. The embodiment of the self in the world suggested by the experiential account is living and being in time and space and the ever-reflexive awareness of meaning and finiteness in the world, expressed by being. This fluid, ever changing account of identity, based on reflexivity and introspection, leaves the self and identity in an isolated position, and to support this James writes that consciousness is a private state of mind and is entirely personal (James, 1890, in 1950 reprint). Whilst this experiential and phenomenological account of identity emphasises personal constructions of experience, owned by the person, a humanist approach focuses on relationships and interpersonal experiences.

### Person-centred psychology

Person-centred psychology was developed in response to critiques of behaviouralism and psychoanalysis. A group of psychologists including Carl Rogers (1951), Eric Fromm (1957) and Abraham Maslow (1965) developed thinking around person-centred encounters, or relationships, as a starting point for understanding. Subjective experience, which means understanding how other people experience themselves, is central to person-centred psychology. Uniqueness and agency of the person are also central concepts of this humanistic approach. Rogers (1951) writes about intersubjectivity as the interaction between two people in understanding the experiences of each other. The uniqueness of the individual in this approach, which includes differences in each person's personal, interpersonal and social experience, can lead to problems in perceiving another person's experience due to interpretation mistakes, according to humanist thinking. The aim of person-centred psychology is to promote the personal unique growth in a self-directed, or agentic, way.

Developments in person-centred thinking have resulted in many wide-ranging methods for use in supporting people in the skills and process of relating to others. In the study included later in this book a person-centred approach to reflexivity and choice of narrative interview methods is taken. The concepts of uniqueness of the person and subjective experience are valuable beginning points for studying the process of identity and that the experience of identity is personal. However, as discussed above, identity is also impacted upon by relationships as well as the wider social world. Tajfel and Turner (1979) incorporate a heavier emphasis on the interaction of the self and the social world in constructing identity.

## Social identity theory

An early, yet still influential, attempt to integrate lived experience from the personal perspective is Tajfel and Turner's work on Social Identity Theory (1979) which sets out a three-stage description of how identity is formed. For them, the three stages of identity formation are social categorisation, social identification and social comparison. In this, social categorisation is based on the cognitive process of categorisation in relation to self-identity. Tajfel and Turner claim that cognitive social categorisation, the first stage, is an everyday mechanism by which people make sense of the social world. The second stage of Social Identity Theory, social identification, takes identity beyond the personal world and typifies the ever-changing identity. At this stage, the social world is acting upon the person's own social categorisation scheme and constantly redefining aspects of identity. The third stage, social comparison, attempts to explain the ways our identities impact on the external social world in the ways we interact with other people. An example of this Social Identify Theory in praxis, which Tajfel and Wilkes (1963) studied extensively, is investigations into racism. Prejudice against other social groups is an example of Social Identity Theory in action. This theory of identity is important as it integrates the cognitive mechanical aspects of a person in respect of categorisation and illustrates how this operates in conjunction with the social world. Here, there are no quantified units of measurement, but conceptual categories that are concerned with meaning.

Whilst Social Identity Theory attempted to explain the connection between personal aspects of identity and the social world, other perspectives have focused on the social world as a starting point for investigation.

## Social perspectives of self

The self as embodied in the social world is traditionally investigated using quantitative methodology. Because of the abstract nature of identity and its inherent components of the self, including consciousness, reflexive awareness, meaning making and autonomy, the quantitative study of identity is problematic (Stephens, 1996). The reliance on accounts of the inner world of the self to explain identity compels these different perspectives to develop with focus on how 'being a person' is expressed. This is done through varying degrees of determination from the external world, and how this expression is embodied within the world. In this sense, the central question in the study of identity is the positioning of the self:

> Here is the problem: do we perceive an ordered world, each from his or her own point of view because we each have an original or native sense of our own singularities? Or do we each have such a sense because we perceive the world in an ordered and centred way? (Harre, 2002, p.73)

The quantification of identity has been investigated empirically through biological and behavioural perspectives in psychology.

### Biological perspectives

The biological perspective, although plagued by the unknown connection between the physical brain and consciousness, is based on the premise that consciousness is an emergent property of the brain (Metcalfe, 2000). In these terms, consciousness is linked to identity through self-awareness; choosing identities and awareness of these identities is linked to conscious awareness of our personal self (Woodward, 2004). Work conducted with people who have experienced brain damage (Metcalfe, 2000) has shown that some cognitive skills are performed outside awareness. It is concluded that, from this biological perspective, consciousness is an innate quality of the brain through the evolutionary process (Metcalfe, 2000). Additionally, with the development of the human large brain in conjunction with the lived experience of an ever more complex social world, the components that contribute to the formation of identity have developed into conscious awareness. These components are consequently expressed through bodily functions as comparative emotions such as fear, pain, happiness, and anger. This embodied self is the pivotal point on which the question of identity hangs due to the presence of both material and socially constructed considerations of the self and the interaction of these in identity construction. In the following sections, an embodied identity and self will be argued for on the basis that (based on the evidence above) both personal and social aspects of the self are necessary to construct identity.

Whilst it is clear that to 'be a person' with an identity, a body is needed, there is some question in psychology and philosophy as to the amount of interaction between consciousness and the body. Whilst the view that the body as a mere vessel ruled by the mind is contested (Yardley, 1997), the methods of investigation into identity and embodiment provide a range of positions as to the role of external influences of society and culture in the formation of identity. In the biological model, embodiment occurs through the sensory system and prescribes the self as almost a 'social dope' that takes in information through the senses, processes this cognitively and churns out appropriate responses (Wetherell & Maybin, 1996). The level of determination of the self in the biological model is high, with a reliance on Darwin's (1859) theory of evolution to explain behaviour through inherited genes. For example, Dawkins' 1993 notion of the selfish gene suggests that the genetic structure of a person dictates that the optimal goal for that person is to perpetuate the gene coding to the next generation, at any cost, and that the basis of behaviour is around this goal. However, certain human social behaviour, such as altruism, cannot be explained in these terms. Altruism, that is, behaviour that serves at a cost to the altruist, would disadvantage the survival of the gene in mating terms. The fact that altruistic behaviour survives in humans and has not evolved out as genetic disadvantage casts some doubt on this purely biological perspective of identity formation.

## Behavioural perspectives

Behavioural perspectives of identity are based on the premise that 'I am what I do' and look to behaviour in the social world to explain identity. In behavioural psychology, experiments are conducted in controlled settings to test and support previously defined categories of social behaviour.

These are based on attributes of that behaviour and aim to quantify the interaction between the embodied self and the social and cultural world in a cause and effect manner. However, some of these studies (Duncan, 1979; Millgram, 1963) have been criticised for use of deception and manipulations that contravene the BPS (1978) guidelines on research using human participants. It is highly doubtful that in a manipulative situation such as deception, the rationale of the experiment or indeed the stressful nature of the experiment would have left the participants unchanged psychologically. This is an important criticism that illustrates the objective nature of cause and effect studies of isolated aspects of behaviour, and the treatment of the person as a variable of the experiment.

The biological and the behavioural perspectives on the nature of the self and formation of identity has its roots in traditional positivist and modernist methods (Gergen, 1991). The epistemological nature of positivist method is that of progress and building on existing knowledge, and although emergent in nature, focuses on a cause and effect functional progression (Danermark et al., 2002). However, it is important, if we are to study identity, to include a personal perspective in order to contextualise identity within society.

## Social construction and the postmodern self

One qualitative method of investigating the self and identity that acknowledges the importance of the social world and its impact on identity is the socially constructed perspective. This socially constructed account of identity in psychology has been investigated using qualitative methods such as discourse analysis. Discourse analysts claim that social constructions of the self are:

> ...continually shaped and reshaped through interactions with others and involvement in social and cultural activities (Wetherell & Maybin, 1996, p.220)

and that

> ...language is not a transparent medium for conveying thought, but actually constructs the world and the self in the course of its use. (Wetherell & Maybin, 1996, p.220).

Whilst acknowledging the experiential position and the importance of reflexive awareness, social constructionists argue that the self is positioned in the social world and is affected by meaning and representations. 'Language' as referred to in the quote above concerns not only spoken language but also semiotics, symbolism, ritual and cultural practice. Gergen (1991) provides an illustration of how the postmodern social constructionist view has developed over time from romanticism, through modernism, to postmodernism.

> Postmodernism seems to the romanticist little short of nihilism: all intrinsic properties of the human being, along with moral worth and personal commitment are lost from view, leaving nothing to believe in. Similarly, the modernist reviles the romanticist for sentimentalism, head-in-the sand impracticality, and the replacement of objective decision making by highfalutin morality, while decrying postmodernism's threats to truth and objectivity. (Gergen, 1991, p.229)

Gergen's analysis of the emergent periods of romanticism, modernism and postmodernism are based upon the cumulative effects of language through time in constructing the social world. Gergen claims that the construction of the self through language depends upon the state of society and culture, and that through various periods (romantic, modern and postmodern) are historically cumulative in their effects on language. This includes the process of science, and in Gergen's view, empirical science is a modernist concept due to its rigid search for universal truth and the consequent modernist commitment to a coherent identity. Conversely, postmodernism has emerged from modernity due to the saturation of society by science and technology, leaving a fragmented identity, parts of which play varying roles as demanded by an ever crowded social world. Consequently, postmodern identity is fluid and ever changing, constructed by language and representations in the saturated social world and therefore relational to the fluid events of the social world. Gergen does not suggest that these periods of history cancel each other out, but that postmodernism embraces them and combines these and other aspects of meaning along with current and future developments.

In support of this, Gergen cites the rapid developments of technology as impacting on identity, for example, the internet and advertising. In the case of both, representations from society are said to shape identity by offering almost unlimited choices in the creation of the self, and the increase of studies into the online virtual identity support this (see for example Leung, 2003).

Gergen points out that the availability of more advanced technological representations provide many more possible internalised, meaning-making examples of potential contributions to the constructions of identity. The availability of more examples of identity facilitates the possibility of a wider range of identities to be constructed, for example, work identity, family role identity and student identity are all identity possibilities for a person to consider. In the course of a day, an individual may interchange between these fragmented identities as, through postmodernism, more diverse and wide-ranging identity opportunities are available.

To sum up Gergen's position, the socially constructed self is fluid and dependent on representations from society and conversations with others that are internalised, reflected upon and embodied in our actions in the world, and most importantly, the meanings we attach to these internal and external dialogues.

Harre (1994) shares Gergen's view when he discusses the time we spend in dialogue with ourselves, and others. Harre suggests that even when we are alone and not in interaction with the world or others, the inner dialogue goes on constructing the identity through conversation with the self. For Harre, the meaning-making nature of this constant dialogue whether with the self, others or the social world is an ongoing process, bringing ever new and changing concepts into conscious awareness. The study of the nature of consciousness is central to Harre's theory of socially constructed identity. Harre (2002) comments:

> Roughly one might say that common to many puzzles about consciousness is the thought that human beings, at least, are aware that they are aware of material things, some of the states of their own body, and can monitor themselves thinking about these and other matters. (Harre, 2002, p.1)

Socially constructed concepts of the self and identity, then, can be illustrated as a constant flow of dialogue between the self and the social world, and the self's awareness and reflection on this. If this interactive identity, with the internal self and the external self constantly communicating with the social world, is to be studied, a person-centred methodology that draws out an account of the inner self, the external self and how the social world has affected the identity is needed. Taking into account then the ever-fluid concept of identity through the construction of social experience, representations of the self through communication processes in terms of socially embedded representations and discourses are discussed next.

## Language and social construction

Whilst there are many ways in which communication between people occurs, with or without words, the conversations we hold with each other are very common form of communication. Not only does language have a rule-based grammar and set of letters and words, but the meanings attached to language and the way it is used in the social situation not only allows for communication between people, but also for the construction of shared object concepts.

However, the socially constructed self, with its completely relativist position, is problematic due to its claims to truth and knowledge and, conversely, the argument against relativism that, if all knowledge and truth are relative, then upon what grounds does the relativist suggest we accept relativism? (Sayer, 2000). An explanation of this argument has been taken up by philosophers as follows. Harre extends Shotter's (1997) joint action theory and his explanation of the construction of lived experience through language. Here, Harre (1992) provides a critique of Gergen's:

> ...extreme form of anti-realism. (Harre, 1992 p.154).

Harre suggests that underlying social constructions are realist notions of conversation, which he describes a joint action, being a necessary property of language exchange, and therefore not relative:

> The one shared thesis is this: all psychological phenomena *and the beings in which they are realised* are produced discursively. Since there could be no being which is both atomic and capable of the intentional use of symbols, the discursive thesis entails a sociality thesis. All action meaningful as acts, that is, action which is capable of sustaining some psychological phenomenon such as remembering or deciding, is joint action. (Harre, 1992, p.154)

Here Harre is defending the embodied aspect of the social world involved in the construction of social construction, since without the exchange of language and other agentic acts of reasoning, social construction cannot occur and therefore the act of conversation must occur and is not a social construction in itself.

Taking into consideration the possibility of many and varied socially constructed fragmented identities and the importance of language in the social construction of identity, the following sections will argue for the existence of a health identity. In addition to this, a suitable methodology for the study of the construction of health identity will be considered.

## Why health identity?

Given the possibility of the self as containing many fragmented identities, and the importance of health discussed in previous chapters of this book, health identity emerges as an important consideration for lived experience. Other important identities, all of which may interact with health identity are gendered identity, racial identity and class identity. In the construction of the self, it becomes clear that these fragmented identities do not appear as discreet identities, but are interactive, explaining the importance of a critical investigation into identity in the context of society.

As discussed in Chapter 1, health is a gendered concept and women's health is defined in a way that reflects both specific reproductive and general health in the context of material health and health experiences. Women's reproductive and general health conceptions are:

> Located firmly within their experience of everyday community living. (Sixsmith & Boneham, 2003, p.239)

Identity concerns self-awareness which includes awareness of the body and of experience in the world. Concepts of health for women include medicalised aspects of material health such as pregnancy, menstruation and menopause in addition to personal and vicarious experiences of health, including social health issues such as being treated for an illness at a hospital or visiting a doctor. Therefore, this identification with health in both social and personal terms provides unique health awareness based on health experiences and provides a health identity. A critical approach to understanding women's health identity is useful as many other aspects of identity interact with health identity. Issues such as racial and cultural identity, gendered identity and class identity integrate with health identity and position the fragmented identity in the range of social possibility and opportunity. Conversely, factors in society, such as media advertising and governmental policy, which are largely out of the control of the individual, may also interact with the fragmented identity in shaping health identity. It is important here to note that the factors that are out of control of the individual can shape identity in both a positive and a negative manner. For example, intervention into health by policy advising better nutrition can positively enhance health for those who take up government advice and build it into their everyday dietary practices; conversely, advertising in the media, which provides normalised images of super-slender women, can be oppressive and contribute to eating disorders (Wilcox & Laird, 2000).

In order to safeguard health and wellbeing it is important for women (and men) to construct their health identity in a way that is fluid, as time is transitional and the ageing body and unique experiences of the world provide challenges to health. This interaction with the world is important for identity construction and particularly for health identity because of material aspects of illness, their visibility to the external world and the lack of control over illness by the individual. The experience of physiological illness is also important as aspects of nursing and care by family or health professionals requires an interaction of health identity and experience with another person in the social world, creating a health relationship. This inevitably involves an embodiment of health in the world, an important aspect of health identity and the process that links the personal to the social.

As can be seen from the widely differing models of identity discussed above, theory is divided in its positioning of the conscious self in terms of determination and agency of the person in creating identity. The consideration of the embodied self-taking action in the world cannot be ignored, and research into identity often has to combine different theories when applying them to what it means to 'be a person' in the world.

## Embodiment and health identity

Embodiment, then, can be seen as a link between the self and the social world in terms of how identity or identities are constructed. In lived experience, many different social situations are encountered and each of these situations is socially and culturally positioned. In order to feel comfortable with the social world, attempts are made to 'fit in' with the variety of available social and cultural positions through, for example, wearing certain clothes or acting in a certain way. In fact, in certain social and cultural positions it becomes morally or legally unacceptable to defy cultural and social 'rules' making these social and cultural positions an imposition (Weber, 1962). By living in the world and encountering social and cultural situations, each person is, to one degree or another, internalising the experience of this. In turn, preferences are developed and expectations realised and these become part of our internal identity. However, this internal identity is not solely influenced by any external force.

Our own emotions also contribute to the construction of our inner identity, as in Harre's (1992) comment that inner dialogue goes on constructing the identity through dialogue. In turn, this inner dialogue contributes to the agentic decisions made to act on the world. Acting on the world, then, involves the material body in the form of physical actions in conjunction with a discursive element which holds the 'embodied conversation' with the social world. This is particularly pertinent in the study of health and health identity, because the concept of health embraces not only physiological health and physical illness but also the health behaviour and attitudes and feelings of every person. Therefore it is crucial that embodiment, in this sense, is investigated.

People living with physical illness experience a full range of identity disruption. Bridgens (2004) explains this in relation to the effects of the experience of polio on the identity of people with polio and post-polio syndrome. She found that acknowledgement of their illness was built into the identity in order to deal with challenging situations that were faced on a day-to-day basis. Not only do they have to take into account their internal identity, the 'I' modified in terms of feelings and emotions such as pain and fear they also have to (sometimes outside their control) embody their health behaviour in the social world. Conversely, the concept of health includes wellbeing, and strategising towards wellbeing necessarily involves constant monitoring of the physical body in conjunction with gathering information from the social world about best practice. It is clear, then that the material body and the discursive self, in reflexive conversation with the social world, constitute a more holistic interaction of identity construction.

**Material bodies and discursive identities**

When considering a model of identity in which the material body interacts with the discursive self, it has been necessary to deconstruct the concept of the material body as the Cartesian concept of an objective vessel. Traditional dualist models depict the body as a physical machine that is ruled by a mind that controls its action (Yardley, 1997). However, Merleau-Ponty (1945) asserts that:

> ...'living' (leben) is a primary process from which, as a starting point, it becomes possible to 'live' (erleben) this or that world, and we must eat or breath before perceiving and awakening to relational living, belonging to colours and lights through sight, to sounds through hearing, to the body of another through sexuality, before arriving at the life of human relations. Thus sight, hearing, sexuality, the body are not the only routes, instruments or manifestations of personal existence: the latter takes up and absorbs into itself their existence as it is anonymously given. (Merleau-Ponty, 1945, p.160)

Merleau-Ponty considers the embodied self, including the material body and the socially constructed identity to be mutually necessary for living and being. As Yardley (1997) observes:

> Indeed, Merleau-Ponty (1945) stands realism on its head by asserting that our physical being is an embodiment of our will to exist, and that embodied selfhood is an accomplishment actively main-

> tained by processes which range from the biological to the psychosocial. (Yardley, 1997, p.10)

As a consequence of this, embodied lived experience can be seen to be meaningful and purposive (Yardley, 1997) and this holistic model negates the realist, positivist paradigm of the objective body separated from the subjective mind. A focus on the corporeal body in medicine and the shortcomings of this has prompted studies into embodiment and its consequences for health. Radley (2000), in a study into the consequences of embodiment for health psychology, states that:

> ...knowledge of the body as object – even when taken across a range of interventions and diagnostic categories – does not itself add up to any adequate understanding of what illness means in a world of embodied persons. (Radley, 2000, p.298)

Radley argues that the body is ever present in health and that health behaviour is constructed in discourse, but that does not mean that the embodied self is constructed solely in discourse. Radley's view that 'doing the body in talk is not the same as acting with the body' (Radley, 2000, p.299) is important, as this critiques the relativist position of health behaviour and includes a realist aspect of the material body. As pointed out in the previous chapter, Cartesian dualist positions in regard to health have prevented the problem of 'body as object' being overcome. Wilde (1999), in a consideration of Cartesian dualism and embodiment, concludes that:

> ...embodiment is not a theory or a group of theories, but a different way of thinking about and knowing human beings. (Wilde, 1999, p.25)

Arguments in favour of taking into account embodiment in health make strong statements about praxis. As qualitative study and critical health psychology has progressed, the study of embodiment has moved away from theory and has been applied to areas such as the birth experience and nursing, where direct contact with healthcare occurs. Showing how the experience of healthcare is inherently connected with issues of embodiment, Goldberg (2002), in a paper about perinatal nursing, comments that:

> ...women and their newborns are discharged home with minimal information and support from health care professionals, and an

> increased reliance on technology, have led to a dehumanisation of the birthing experience. The manner in which women are treated and cared for leaves many women with a sense of alienation and disconnection from their bodies. (Goldberg, 2002, p.446)

This is a clear example of the social impact of objectification of the body. Chater examines the experiences of older people within health-care and found that the ageing experience was 'a reflexive interplay between discourse, body and a history of the present' (Foucault, 1978; Chater, 2002). In addition to this, Chater's findings show that older people often interpret the body as 'other', dissociating themselves from the part of the body that was 'ill'. Illness and ageing then, according to Chater, are bound up with internal discourses, material body and discourse in society.

It is clear from the studies above that there is an increased need to consider embodiment in any study of identity and particularly health identity. Social science, then needs to:

> Confront the question of how the social realm itself is embodied: a notion which can give form to the relationship between the social structural milieu in which humans live, their subjective experience and the flesh through which that existence is lived. (Lyon, 1996, p.69)

This fluid health identity that internalises the societal narrative of health and embodies the personal health narrative in the world is continually constructed, then, in a lived existence of time and location. If health experience is to be treated subjectively and holistically in terms of embodiment, attention must be given to how a health identity is constructed over a period of time.

## Investigating health identity construction in terms of embodiment

As can be seen by the widely differing perspectives on conscious awareness and identity construction presented above, neither the quantification of objective concepts of identity nor the consideration of the qualitative subjective aspects of identity provide a satisfactory explanation of what 'being a person' is like in the world. Issues of embodiment, of the material self and the discursive self make acknowledgement of both the physical body and socially constructed society in the formation of an identity imperative. When considering health identity, this consideration becomes even more pertinent. In the context of both wellbeing and illness, encompassing not only physical aspects of biological illness and wellbeing, but also emotional responses and attitudes to being well or being ill, these are consequently embodied in the social world as health behaviour.

Discursive aspects of the self are integral in the construction of identity. Therefore, in order to investigate identity construction, the discursive or narrative self must be clarified.

## The narrative self

The biological and behavioural perspectives on models of identity formation are largely concerned with the objective investigation of measurable ingredients that make up a solid model of identity and the remixing of these ingredients to form categories into which identity, and consequently people, are neatly compartmentalised. However, the social world is not as simplistic as this. In lived experience, a person recognises aspects of identity through subjective awareness. Emotions such as fear, happiness, anger and pain are experienced internally and embodied in behaviour and communication in the social and cultural world. In acknowledging this, problems of the subjective nature of identity raise parallel problems of the study of identity. If the study of identity is to be taken out of the controlled objective measurement oriented environment of traditional scientific methods, what are the ontological and epistemological implications for the study of identity?

Ontologically, what is being studied moves from the quantification of an object to the breadth and depth of the quality of an abstract subject. Because of the fluidity of the abstract identity, the epistemological base of traditional science (i.e. building on the blocks of previous knowledge to find or support a truth) is shifted to the fluidity and therefore the relativity of an ever-changing social world (Gergen, 1991). In everyday experience, making sense of the world depends heavily on both introspection of identity and the embodiment of this identity through our actions on the world. In turn, the social and cultural aspects of the world around us impact on our identity through a multitude of representations presented to us and experienced by us. Throughout our lives, this unique cumulative effect of subjective experience is built into 'what being is like' for us. The uniqueness of these interactive combinations is personally relative to each person, and this enables us to make sense of an ever-changing world and act as an autonomous agent on that world. Consequently, because our relative combination of experience is different from another person's relative experiences, what is true is also relative from the personal perspective.

Therefore, from an epistemological point of view, to gather accounts from the subjective perspective of lived experience will give a more transparent view of how identity is formed than attempting to find a universal truth through traditional scientific methods. The investigation of this subjective experience in the context of society is absent from the perspectives above. However, narrative psychology provides an opportunity to study personal accounts of lived experience.

### The narrative self and storytelling

The narrative self appears as the construction of a story that spans the temporal base of a lifetime connecting the personal self with the social self from past to lived present and on to anticipated future. The difference between the narrative self and other versions of studies of the self as critiqued above are that the narrative self is a part of the self that is brought about through self-awareness in order to interact with the social world through itself as narration. As Ricoeur (1985) comments:

> Without the recourse to narration, the problem of personal identity would in fact be condemned to an antimony with no solution. Either we must posit a subject identical with the self through the diversity of its different states, or, following Hume and Nietzsche, we must hold that this identical subject is nothing more than a substantial illusion, whose elimination brings to light a pure manifold of cognitions, emotions, a violation. (Ricoeur, 1985, p.246)

The narrative self, then, takes a position of claiming this storied identity and recounting reflexively on the constructed experience of the self. In contrast to the self as an object for study by someone in the context of a discreet subject, the narrative self is positioned as an opportunity to report on the unique, fluid construction of experience in the context of a life. Ricoeur goes on to explain:

> Unlike the abstract identity of the Same, the narrative identity, constitutive of self constancy, can include change, mutability, within the cohesion of one lifetime. The subject appears both as reader and writer of its own life, as Proust would have it. As the literary analysis of autobiography confirms, the story of a life continues to be refigured by all the truthful or fictive stories a subject tells about

> himself, or herself. This refiguration makes this life itself a cloth woven of stories told. (Ricoeur, 1985, p.246)

Ricoeur continues to explain that self-constancy constitutes a reflexive account of life filtered through social and cultural experiences which are present in the narrative account of the self.

A critique of life as narrative is that lived experience often does not travel in a linear temporal direction, and is chaotic. Whilst this is true, and the self is often in crisis and confusion, Frank (2000a) explains that the narrative self brings meaning-making and change to chaotic lived experience, and the narrative self is able to reflexively prioritise temporal aspects of the self so as to understand lived experience. Frank (2000a) approaches the illness narrative from the postmodern position of the person who is ill 'reclaiming the authority and ability to tell his or her story' (Frank, 2000a, p.171), a position which fits with the aims of the exploration of health identity.

By illustrating the modernist position of the ill person being 'colonised' by medicalisation, Frank contrasts the discourse of the medical patient with the discourse of the ill person. Frank's work on illness focuses on four themes of illness narrative: the restitution narrative, the chaos narrative, the quest narrative and the testimony narrative.

Sustaining the identity is an important part of identity construction that is tracked by the narrative. In illness narratives, disjoins (McAdams, 1993) and narrative wreckage (Frank, 2000a) are common and the continuum of the identity is problematic. These narrative wreckage and disjoins are points in accounts where major changes and perhaps traumatic events turn the narrative account away from the original plot and often onto a different trajectory. Study of the ill person's narrative away from the methodological structure of the medical world uncovers the meaning and experience of the ill person, removed from the illness discourse.

Roberts (2003) explains that these attempts to bring order out of the chaotic lived experience results in the telling of the story, or it's emplotment, in a relatively, but often not completely, ordered fashion. As we do this on an internal level on an everyday basis, the narrated autobiographical account recounts this to the outside world. Building on this, a relatively new approach that investigates narrative identity and the narrative self is narrative psychology. Crossley (2000b) states:

> The aim of narrative psychology is therefore to study the language, stories and narratives which constitute selves and the implications

> and permutations of those narratives for individuals and societies. (Crossley, 2000b, p.40)

Narrative psychology uses qualitative methods such as interviews to obtain personal accounts of the narrative self from people around a particular phenomenon. Narrative psychology has much in common with social constructivist and discourse analysis approaches as the use of language in narrative psychology is inherently linked with meaning-making and consequently identity construction (Crossley, 2000a).

The narrative approach uses a person-centred account of lived experience to investigate identity by attempting to draw out a coherent account of the inner self and how this self is represented in the ideological and positioned external world. Dan McAdam's (1993) proposed a model of narrative inquiry, which, by designing an interview schedule that elicited an account in story form, would encourage the participant to explain not only their personal views and opinions, but place these in the context of societal and cultural issues. In contrast to discourse analysis, where the focus is on the text, narrative inquiry looks at lived experience, taking into account temporal aspects of the self in terms of the lifespan (Greene, 2000). Narrative enquiry typically deals with whole life accounts of experience, which allows the historical, social and cultural issues of the narrative self to emerge, in addition to any current emotions that relate to these issues. The narrative self as explained by a narrative enquiry is not solely an explanation of the inner self, but also explains interaction with the social, moral, cultural and political groundings of the self in society. This gives valuable insight into how the self is embodied in the social world and how the social world impacts on the self through the analysis of symbols and discourse through the imagery contained in the narrative account. This methodology makes the task of investigating the process of interaction in the construction of identity possible as it takes into account, from a subjective perspective, various aspects of the fluid self, including embodiment. Critical health psychology and the interactive nature of the inner self with the external world through discourse and narrative inevitably involves the body as a medium for communication. Frank (2000a) comments that:

> Bodies are realised – not just represented but created – in the stories they tell. This realisation can and should be reflexive: by telling certain stories, ethical choices are made; the choices in turn generate stories. Common sense understands people as having some responsibility for their stories and for their bodies. Common sense is less accustomed to the possibility of exercising that responsibility for bodies through

> stories. One road to the achievement of the communicative body is though storytelling. (Frank, 2000a, p.52)

Embodiment, therefore, particularly in health identity as where considerations of the corporeal body are included in health identity, is a vital link in understanding identity construction.

The study included in this book, then, is based on the premise that there is not a single personal identity, separate from the social world, but that identity is fluid and constantly interactive *with* the social world. This is clearly a two-way conversation, as to live in the social world not only do we embody ourselves, but we also internalise, through the perceptions of our material body, the world into ourselves in the process of identity construction.

In the study included in this book the personal health identity construction of women will be investigated through narrative accounts. These narrative accounts will expose, through symbols and images contained within the account, an account of self as embodied in the social world, and how this interacts with identity formation. The study is also designed to draw out accounts of which institutional-based social representations of health are obtained by the women taking part in order to investigate health identity as represented in the social world.

## Social theory and locating identity in society

So far we have looked at personal perspectives of identity study and how these relate to the social world. In the next chapter, the social world and where personal identities fit into society will be explored. This is to clarify the important role of the context of society in the construction of identity. As discussed above, personal identity and interpersonal identity is impacted upon by the social world. As discussed earlier politicised aspects of society such as gender, class, ethnicity and economic status influence the construction of identity and in particular women's identity. The location of women in society and the way their identity is constructed is a project for feminism.

## Conclusion: The story so far

The explanation of the construction of a health identity in this chapter has shown that identity formation is:

- Fluid and ongoing
- Gendered

- Embodied in society
- Fragmented within postmodern identity
- Narrated in everyday talk

A further area of study has taken this issue of objectification of women and gendered health and moved the investigation to a deeper level of analysis: why have women been objectified? The patriarchal nature of gendered health is well documented (Ussher, 2000; Yardley, 1997) and the societal discourses of gender politics have been of interest to feminist study.

Gendered health and societal discourses often have negative effects on women's self image, throwing their identity into crisis. Theorists (for example De Beauvoir, 1949) commented that identity does not become an issue until it is questioned, until 'the other' is recognised. Feminist researchers have taken up this crisis of identity and in observing women as 'the other' in society have theorised the impact and possible solution to this disruption of women's identity. In light of the above consideration, the next chapter considers the power dynamics with the aim of assessing the effects of feminist theory and patriarchal health representations as competing theoretical discourses available in society on the identity construction of women. As health includes not only experience but also the material body, a feminist standpoint will be considered as an appropriate landscape for health identity construction.

# 4
# Feminist as Far as Possible – The Feminist Health Identity and Critical Realism

## Introduction

This book focuses on the lived experience of women and the construction of their health identity. In this chapter, arguments around how feminist identity impacts on women's identities is taken into account and if this has, in fact, changed the way that women live in society is investigated. Also, because women's lives are positioned in the embodied lived experience, a critical realist framework is appropriate. Critical realism and aspects of narrative truth are also explored later in this chapter. Initially, the position of women in relation to health identity and society will be discussed.

## Woman as 'other'

Identity theories suggest that the social world is a mirror in which we constantly look to construct our identity in a changing and fluid way (Mead, 1934). If the social world remains stable then identity continues to construct itself in the same way causing no cause for concern. Conversely, if the social world becomes challenging, and alternative available identities are observed, then we encounter a time when the social world does not reflect who we think we are and our identity changes, either willingly or through shaping by society. However, this identification with difference, perhaps resulting in an 'identity crisis', does not operate solely on a personal and interpersonal level (Woodward, 2004). The feminist project has recognised that patriarchy has become institutionalised and the oppression of women is a personal problem, not just one of political theory. In terms of this, the most appropriate approach for the current study is feminist standpoint theory, which values difference within difference (or the individual uniqueness and equality of the person) and, when underpinned by a critical realist approach to health, acknowledges woman's material body in feminist theory.

Gergen (1999) explains this identification with difference in terms of 'identity politics' and 'relational theory'. Gergen suggests that Western thought on identity is individualistic, and that the theory of the socially constructed identity and it's involvement in identity politics, although seemingly interactive, is based on the personal and does not take into account the interpersonal nature of identity. Gergen explains that the basis of the problem is:

> To appreciate the blossoming of relational theory, consider a long-standing intellectual problem the significance of which is matched only by its resistance to solution: how is interpersonal understanding achieved – how do we comprehend others' meanings (or fail to do so)? (Gergen, 1999, p.6)

Gergen critiques the premise that the socially constructed identity is constructed in the individual mind, and argues that identity politics, based on this, becomes redundant to relational politics. Identity politics involves the proposal that excluded politically active groups constitute their identity from the individual identities of the group members. These excluded groups are typically groups that are oppressed by an inherent characteristic that is naturally produced and unchangeable such as race or sex. The socially constructed standpoint is taken up by identity politics due to the emancipatory nature of social constructions within the groups towards the common good, or equality. The empirical paradigm, which followed a fixed path of pre-designated patriarchal knowledge and truth production, is abandoned for the possibility of 'something new and different'. However, by assuming that identity is personal in the first place and that all concepts are constructed in discourse, Gergen suggests that:

> The prevailing rhetoric has been of little influence outside groups of the already committed. For the targets – those most in need of 'political education' – such rhetoric has more often been alienating and counter-productive. By and large identity politics has depended on a rhetoric of blame, the illocutionary effects of which are designed to chastise the target (for being unjust, prejudiced, inhumane, selfish, oppressive, and/or violent). In Western culture we essentially

> inherit two conversational responses to such forms of chastisement – incorporation or antagonism. (Gergen, 1999, p.2)

Here Gergen argues that the identity formation of the group and the consequent rhetoric produced are based in an individualistic rhetoric of the group members without taking into account the dialectical position of the 'target'. Barker (1999) sums this up by stating that:

> Collective subject positions are always socially constructed and partial. Therefore, although the need for political solidarity to combat oppression has never been greater, that solidarity must acknowledge the partial and contradictory construction of subjects. (Barker, 1999, p.107)

This has been a problem for the feminist project, and partially explains why women today, in praxis, may be no more equal than the women of Simone De Beauvoir's France of 1949.

It would be useful at this point to look briefly at the history of feminist theory in terms of progress made by way of relational identity and to see how women, who have recognised that they are perceived as 'other' by patriarchal society, have dealt with the ensuing crisis of identity.

## Working backwards – Historical aspects of feminist theory

Men and women have, since records began, been treated as different from each other. The difference in the sexual reproductive organs of male and female human beings (De Beauvoir, 1949) is the realist reasoning behind this differentiation, although this essentialism does not account for the repercussions for women in terms of societal and cultural issues. Much of feminist study has focused on inequalities in general and particularly those involving women's health and the impact which women's social roles, cultural context and discursive representations have upon women's health (Ussher, 2000).

The development of feminist thought has emerged as a response to the recognition of inequalities of power within a patriarchal society, beginning with early feminist thought and first wave radical feminism which was iconised by Sojourner Truth and the Suffrage Movement. Eventually women were given the right to vote in Britain in 1928. Feminist theory was advanced by De Beauvoir in 1949. De Beauvoir examined the biological, historical and mythical roles of women in society in addition to the adolescent, adult, situational and liberationary roles of women in lived experience.

Second Wave Feminism emerged and it became clear that any equality would be in the light of an admission that there was something to be equal to; a male supreme 'norm' to which women must strive for equality. Researchers therefore studied difference between the genders (Stainton-Rodgers & Stainton-Rodgers, 2001) and focused on the emphasis of the unique strengths of women within the patriarchal society.

Some feminists began to realise that within feminism some women were 'more equal' than others. With the recognition of women's differences from men, and their unique strengths, multidimensions of discrimination were highlighted. For example, white middle class British women would have fewer problems ignoring the political and financial oppression of patriarchal society than a woman of colour living in poverty in USA, with no social security system and four small children (Crowley & Himmelweit, 1992).

## Feminism, postmodernism, and the development of the feminist standpoint

The individual social context of a woman's life became the postmodern currency for the feminist examination of difference within difference (Wilkinson, 1996) and Foucault's abandonment of the grand narrative (Foucault, 1978) provided a theoretical backdrop for feminist standpoint theory to deconstruct discourse and interrogate socially constructed identity. The recognition that actual women's lives and their experiences, which are inseparable from the political and economic hegemonic factors which influence them, 'are not necessarily the same as feminist knowledge of women's lives' (Hennessey, 1995, p.3), prompted an advanced enquiry into how feminism and women's lives are linked.

Hennessey (1995) examines how postmodernism and the socially constructed world provide a critique of feminism as a counter-hegemonic ideology. Hennessey argues that in modern discourse feminism positions itself with an empirical group identity, generalising itself to all women irrespective of their socio-political circumstances. Feminist standpoint theory, however, provides a way of reconciling women's lives with feminist knowledge. This, according to Harding, is effected by deconstructing the feminist group identity organised around the grand narrative of unity which should be strived for by women and reconstructing feminism to incorporate all socio-political struggles which are inclusive in the standpoint of all women's in their struggles for fairness and equality (Harding, 1986). Harraway (1991) investigates the feminist standpoint perspective on the construction of scientific knowledge and concludes that:

> Feminism is, in part, a project for the reconstruction of public life and public meanings; feminism is therefore a search for new stories, and so for a language which names a new vision of possibilities and limits. (Harraway, 1991, p.25)

This feminist epistemology examines how women (and other marginalised groups) can gain privileged knowledge through practice and struggle. Similarly, Harstock (1999) explains how gender is a divide along which this privileged knowledge can be generated. The additional perspective of women who have lived as marginalised groups through economic, social and political misogynistic practices, provides for the development not only of masculine knowledge but also of the knowledge of the lived experience of the marginalised group. This privileged knowledge, according to Hennessey, allows analysis of gender as constructed in discourse and practice, including misogyny. For example:

> Thinking of heterosexuality as one of the nodal points in the interdiscourse of capitalist-patriarchal gender ideology makes it possible to address the ways 'the regulatory fiction of sexual coherence' is written into the cultures as a way of making sense of sex difference. Heterosexuality depends on the assumption that sex differences are binary opposites and the simultaneous equation of this sex difference with gender. (Hennessey, 1995, p.15)

This example of how sex differences are constructed and idealised is an example of a model of how women's lives can be understood in terms of knowledge through the interrogation of the socially constructed and discursive standpoints of women. Assumptions about sex differences generated through narratives over time and the misogynistic and patriarchal society in feminist standpoint theory critiques are deeply embedded as interpreted in society through gender stereotyping (Ussher, 1991).

In terms of stereotyping of gendered health, women's bodies had become objectified and medicalised to the extent that her body was illustrated in literature and in the structure of society as a collection of reproductive organs that were 'not male' (De Beauvoir, 1949). Foucault's argument that:

> The Mother, with her negative image of 'nervous woman', constituted the most visible form of the hysterisation. (Foucault, 1978, p.74)

criticises the structural nature of science and medicine, particularly psychoanalysis, as this is a clear example of the power of the patriarchal society and the hegemonic male identity subordinating women (Courtenay, 2000).

Current thinking on the feminist standpoint is outlined and revised by Harstock (1999). Harstock explains the link between Marxist theory and feminist theory. Using the Marxist model of the privileged standpoint of the proletariat (Marx, 1954) Harstock attempts to extend Marx's class theory to embrace the work of women and consequently the sexual labour divide into a feminist theory. However, Harstock is explicit about the limitations of postmodernism thought, where action is reduced to discourse and all is relative, commenting that:

> Postmodern theories, I have held, represent the situated knowledge's of a particular social group – European, American, masculine and racially as well as economically privileged. (Harstock, 1999, p.251)

It is in this context that Harstock criticises postmodernism, as feminism so clearly includes all women, and, more specifically, women outside the particular social group stated above. Harstock instead borrows the dialectical and historical materialism of Marxist theory as realist concepts. This allows for the feminist standpoint to be grounded in the everyday experiences of women dominated by capitalist and, more particularly, patriarchal power structures. Importantly, Harstock's work is developed directly from her experiences as a feminist activist. However, dialectical thinking involves:

> ...mode of understanding provides a means for us to investigate the manifold ways social forces are related, a way to examine a world in which 'objects' are defined by the relations coming to focus in them, and in which these objects are constantly chan-

ging in response to the weights of other factors. (Harstock, 1999, p.93)

Therefore, Harstock's feminist standpoint endorses a socially constructed social world that in turn acknowledges the intransience of the acceptance of human activity as ontology. This is not unlike Harre's (1994) argument that the conversation is the intransient occurrence that facilitates the construction of discourse that, for social constructionists, shapes the social world. Further, Harstock's reliance on historical materialism, where the generation of knowledge is cumulative and evolutionary, grounds ontological and epistemological claims subjectively.

The similar philosophical bases of feminist standpoint theory and critical realism are apparent, in part through their augmentation of Marxist theory, albeit in different directions, but also through the acceptance that although the social world is socially constructed and transiently relative, there are realist, intransient aspects that cannot be ignored. In considering health identity, feminist standpoint theory allows for the study of the experience of a person-defined sex, (intransient in Nature), and by gender, (transient by culture). For women, feminist standpoint theory supports the privileged position. A woman, as part of an oppressed group becoming an ontological subject in her own right, obtains by and through an extended epistemology of experiencing 'being a person' in the oppressed group. Additionally, having knowledge of the oppressor, which by society she is forced to recognise and interact with in order to survive, provides this standpoint. In this project, it remains to be seen how, by studying women's health women are oppressed and empowered by health experiences, and how this is reflected in their health identity. By using the feminist standpoint as a model the experiences of women is the privileged standpoint from which these power dynamics can be exposed, and through dialectical considerations, how women socially construct their own health story to combine, strategise and cope with health considerations.

## Relational gender identity politics

In common with Gergen's relational theory of identity, Butler (1990) used a relational theory of identity and focused on gender. Like

De Beauvoir (1949), Butler's feminist agenda asks the question 'what is woman?' However, Butler comments that:

> The very subject of women is no longer understood in stable or abiding terms. (Butler, 1990, p.1)

Butler takes a critical approach to gender study in that she places gender as a socially constructed performance. In these terms, gender would be largely dependant on cultural, social and political situations of the women involved and would therefore be unique to each woman. This is an important point, as Bulter points out that feminism should not be treated as a group action, but as a project for individual women to take up in lived experience. This is similar to Gergen's argument about the rhetoric of identity politics, where 'targets for blame' are identified by groups who assume a group identity. As Gergen points out, this group mentality is futile without the reinforcement of individual identities to support the action. Butler relocates this in gender study by explaining that by forming feminist groups, women are merely isolating themselves from men, which is a more radical feminist position. In place of this, Butler urges a relational model and recommends that society reconsiders gender roles and makes them accessible for both sexes, negating stereotyped gender roles and making them relational to each social, cultural and political situation that is encountered. This view is similar to that of De Beauvoir (1949) who states that:

> ...it is necessary, for one thing, that by and through their natural differentiation men and women unequivocally affirm their brotherhood. (De Beauvoir, 1949, p.741)

However, gender politics mostly ignore the corporeal body and concentrate on gendered behaviour and notions of gender equality. Further, the body is important in today's world, as discussed in Chapter 3, as how we embody ourselves in the world is a vital part of identity construction. Feminist standpoint and postmodern feminism deals with the theoretical aspects of feminism, which place feminism as part of a larger project of social justice and human rights. Francis comments that:

> Those using the term 'gender' often did so in order to suggest that differences in behaviour according to sex were social, rather than biologically driven, phenomenon. However, this position has been

> queried because the intractable link and theoretical slippage between sex (biological) and gender (social). (Francis, 2002, p.40)

Therefore, when considering lived experience of women today in society, the corporeal body must be included in any feminist examination of identity construction due to the institutional effects of health and health representations in society.

## Women's lives in today's society: Theory into practice – or not?

Despite Margaret Thatcher's statement in 1980 that, 'The battle for women's rights has largely been won!' the oppression of women continues in today's society. The rhetoric of the oppression of women has been transformed over the past two decades to a more politically correct discourse. On one hand, the profile of personal aspects of oppression such as domestic violence and childcare issues has been raised and attempts to address these with zero tolerance policing, flexible working hours and crèche facilities have been made. On the other hand, institutionalised oppression, particularly those institutions grounded heavily in patriarchal control, such as the medical profession and the media, has not made such progress. Such dualities have had the effect that women may think that they are more equal by perhaps paying lip service to equality through rhetorical placating gestures by political organisation, but oppression has become more implicitly disguised.

Issues such as these encountered in everyday life have had a confusing effect on women and with the ever increasing saturation of women's identities by media and technology (Gergen, 1991) presenting more possibilities, women are reaching out towards a glass ceiling which they know they should be able to break through because theory tells them they can, but in practice they cannot. Whilst wanting to be equal and identifying with feminism as an institution which offers this possibility, women query why they encounter difficulties in lived experience concerning equality. Living in oppression whilst being told that you are not is confusing enough in itself; the context of women's lives has expanded not into equality, but often into taking on both the 'roles' of women and of men through the concepts of women's work (in the home) and men's work (outside the home). The institutionalised family has moved on from a traditional hierarchical model of power dynamics. This traditional hierarchical model, which is based on Weber's (1962) authority theory of power, provides an explanatory framework for families' organised in this way. In this idealist model of the family, the power is hierarchical and judgement is deferred to those on a higher level of the hierarchy. However, the crumbling of traditional family values and ideologies has led to a more fragmented organisation of the family, which maps more readily onto Foucault's (1978) model of power where the dynamics of control are fluid and changeable unlike Weber's rigid hierarchical model. Foucault's self-regulatory power expresses the organisation of society as fluid and consequently the postmodern family consists of several different permutations of members, and the power dynamic of the family is not hierarchical, but ever changing according to the competing needs for organisation and control (e.g., financial, emotional). Today's society, with a growing number of single parent families and same sex parents in addition to traditional families, is clearly increasingly postmodern in nature. However, the ideological nature of the hierarchical family still exists in previous generations and these values are still transmitted through generations and permeate today's more fragmented organisational model of the family, causing a crisis in values.

Whilst told that women are equal and respected, everyday life and a more globalised media (Giddens, 1991) confirms that women are still objectified. How a woman embodies herself is still measured on male oriented media expectations (Conboy et al., 1997) and women's wombs are still removed from their bodies to 'cure' PMS and menopause. The baseline for 'what is woman' is anything that men do not view as pathological, and that maximises men's opportunity to achieve their potential, at the cost of women. For example, in the medical model of health HRT is promoted as the 'cure all' for menopausal symptoms. Claims made for HRT by the medical profession include firmer, younger looking skin and alleviations of moodiness (Social Issues Research Centre, 2001). Despite all the risks involved in taking HRT women still take it in order, partially, to conform to the accepted male norm of young, thin, white, smiling women (Conboy et al., 1997) that we find staring from the cover of women's magazines and from our television screens.

We have seen, however, in the introduction that evidence suggests that the menopause is a long-term series of hormonal changes that can take a decade to culminate in the loss of menstruation. Secondly, and more damaging, is the implication of the popular media that a woman's biological clock is linked solely to the menopause, and will have 'finally run down' when the menopause happens. This propagates a very negative concept of post menopausal women. The negative scientific cause and effect paradigm of the menopause is heavily reliant on negative concepts of degradation of the body. Al-Azzawi (1991) describes the menopausal process as:

> The menopause is a consequence of oestrogen deficiency due to the depletion, or relative absence, of primordial follicles responsive to the rising levels of gonadotrophins. This deficiency results in target organ failure, e.g. failure to induce endometrial proliferation and subsequent menstrual bleeding. (Al-Azzawi, 1991, p.262)

This scientific description of the menopause as a consequence of negative events is at odds with the concept of menopause as a positive transition experienced by many women (Komesaroff et al., 1997) as is the contentious idea of the biological clock 'running down' at the time of the menopause.

The biological clock is the idea of the body's circadian, infradian and ultradian rhythms that are symbiotic with the outside environment, for example sleep and seasonal change. On the level of the physiological body, external influences such as light and dark affect interact with the cycles of the internal body on a 24 hour basis. Ultradian rhythms and infradian rhythms serve to create a symbiotic environment for the maintenance of circadian rhythms. However, infradian rhythms are as follows:

> The oestrus cycle modulation of locomotive is an example of an infradian rhythm. Another example would be the 28-day human menstrual cycle. (Toates, 1998, p.251)

It is clear from this explanation of biological clocks that women's reproductive cycles are included in these natural cyclic rhythms but do not encompass them. Some media reports have suggested that the biological clock is hinged on a woman's reproductive cycle; however, if the biological clock (i.e. circadian, infradian and ultradian rhythms) ran down, one would be dying or dead. This negative connotation of women rendered useless after the menopause is common and women are now so afraid of the ageing process that they actively try to reverse it by risky activities such as taking HRT or having plastic surgery (Komesaroff et al., 1997). Because of the competing concepts of what women 'should be' based on the patriarchal model of femininity, the media reinforcement of this, and what women are actually experiencing, women may be experiencing a struggle with identity. This includes the personal lived experience combining physiological health and social effects, the interpersonal effects of male oppression and objectification, and the institutional social constructions of competing grand narratives when constructing identity. It is confusion around these body politics and social politics that throws the identity of women into crisis and raises again the enduring question, 'What is woman?' This brings us back to the issue of the patriarchal institutionalised objectification of women's bodies and how this is represented in society.

**Health and the lived experience: What is 'real' for women?**

The position so far in this book is that in order to study women's health identity, lived experience must be studied. It has been shown that women construct their identity on a relational basis, which involves not just personal interpersonal relationships, but also representations from patriarchal and hegemonic institutions such as the media and the medical model of health. Similarly, feminism has become institutionalised. It is clear that in this complex combination of societal and cultural pressures women are making some headway towards equality in law, but in everyday life problems still remain in the guise of healthcare and entertainment.

This highlights the question of when constructing their health identity, how much of these competing institutionalised representation do women regard as 'real' and internalise into their identity which is embodied in the world? Which, of all the theory and representations available through society, do women turn into praxis in their own lives? Popay et al. comments that the normative referent occurs due to:

> ...potential interactions between individual and collective action which may affect the health of individuals and populations and 'ontological fit' – people's ability to (re) construct a positive identity. (Popay et al., 2003, p.55)

In identity (re)-construction in terms of women's health, the issues of contention are the body, by which the woman embodies herself in the world, and the socially constructed society and culture, which in turn serve as a point of reference for normative health.

Complicating this are the issues of the patriarchal objectification of the corporeal body by the medical model of health and the media, and the competing feminist narrative of equality. To understand how women reconstruct their health identity in the light of impending infertility, taking into consideration the corporeal body, as one must in any study of health (Witz, 2000), and the meaning-making process of socially constructed society and culture and the powerful institutions contained therein, deeper consideration of the realist and the relativist philosophical theories.

Health is a unique area of study in the case of philosophy, because to study health or illness, which are perceived as physiological disorders, a realist stance must be taken. However, to study the effects of a physiological disorder, any psychological or philosophical investigation must go further than the medical model of 'the body as a machine' (Descartes, 1647, in 1969 translation) and aim to evaluate the embodiment of health on a personal and interpersonal level and the resulting health identity. This, as shown previously, is a culmination of various socially constructed ideological positions, resulting in an 'ontological fit' and therefore entirely relational.

Critical realism is a philosophical position that, as its name suggests, takes a starting point of realism and relates this to a relativist construction of the world. The next section will examine what critical realism means for women's health identity and for this study.

## Critical realist philosophy of science – Neither realism nor relativism

Critical realism has emerged as a critique of positivism and Harre (1970) introduced ideas of underlying generative mechanisms, which are processes that link together concepts of realism and relative social constructions. Bhaskar (1978) developed the basis for critical realism and presents a theory of science where the world is structured, differentiated, stratified and changing. In critique of positivism Bhaskar identified:

> ...three ontological domains of reality; the empirical, the actual and the real. The empirical domain consists of what we experience, directly or indirectly. It is separated form the actual domain where events happen whether we experience them or not. What happens in the world is not the same as that which is observed. But this domain is in turn separated from the real domain. In this domain there is also that which can produce events in the world, that which metaphorically can be called mechanisms. (Danermark et al., 2002, p.20)

Bhaskar's critique of positivism and empiricism, where science reduces 'what is' to 'what we can know about it' (Bhaskar, 1978), expands the rationale of scientific work to:

> ...investigate and identify relationships and non-relationships, respectively, between what we experience, what actually happens,

> and the underlying mechanisms that produce the events in the world. (Danermark et al., 2002, p.21)

So, according to Bhaskar, critical realism provides a philosophy of science, which, through differentiation between transive (fluid) and intransive (fixed) objects allows for the identification of ontological domains and epistemological mechanisms. This allows for us to investigate not only the formerly empirical (i.e. observable) properties of reality, but also socially constructed entities (such as society) through the identification of underlying, or 'deep', generative mechanisms. Critical realism has implication for health psychology where the intransive aspects of the material body interact closely with the transive aspects of self and society in context.

## Critical realist health psychology

Certain aspects of the health experience are real, tangible, physiological, objective and generalised to a population. For example, and in particular relevance to this project, the reproductive cycle of women is not just a concept but a physical reality, which requires specific and considerable intervention to alter or stop. This physiological sex-specific circadian rhythm (Toates, 1998) provides a signposting system for the reproductive cycle and future expectation of health on which a woman bases her socially constructed health identity. The menopause, for example, provides a milestone in mid life for women, which is an inevitable sign of loss of fertility. Although the socially constructed experience of perimenopause and menopause are not universally the same for all women (Lock, 1998), the reality of the menopause as complete irreversible loss of fertility is universal throughout all women (Toates, 1998). This is the challenge of an absolute reality, to relativist thought, which is determined by truth being mutable and relative to itself and everything else. In terms of women's health psychology, this challenge applies to the intransive reality of being a woman outside discourse and social construction and the relativist position that allows a woman to be anything she wishes to be.

## Critical realism and social science research

Critical realist rationale on investigations in social science, with the transive, artefactual, ideal and social realms and the intransive material realm impact on critical health psychology by enabling a way to incorporate the investigation of the material bodily experience with the socially constructed health experience. Williams (1999) sums up the contribution of critical realist thinking to health research:

> A critical realist approach, it is suggested, enables us to : (i) bring the biological body, impaired or other wise, 'back in'; (ii) relate the individual to society in a challenging, non-conflationary or non 'unidirectional' way; and (iii) rethink questions of identity, difference and ethics of care through commitment to real bodies and real selves, real lives and real worlds. (Williams, 1999, p.797)

In respect of women's health and this project, the additional problems of the oppression of women by not just the hegemonic male but also by patriarchal organisations (such as medicalised health, the tabloid media and positivist medically influenced women's magazine reporting) can be approached and understood in philosophical terms by looking at critical realism in respect of the dialectical position and the synthesis achieved by negotiation of this dialectical position by construction of a health identity. The dialectical position, endorsed by Bhaskar (1978) involves reciprocal causality as mentioned above where the epistemological knowledge generation becomes the ontological object and exists as a structure independently of the epistemology. This knowledge generation is often expressed as the synthesis between thesis and antithesis in dialectics (Marx, 1954) whereby synthesis is the resulting process between two polar opposites in the dialectic. In general, this negotiation happens on an everyday basis to a greater or lesser extent. However, in relation to the notion of oppression, the ontology of the oppressive theory is reinforced by practical activity and consequently knowledge generation that produces an ever-larger body of theory. Only by dialectical analysis of the power structures to identify conflict, and more importantly, activism to oppose the oppressor can the generation of knowledge, influence the ontology of oppression and equate the balance of power. An example of this is the complex power dynamic between institutions such as feminism, health agencies and the media and how this has served to influence lived experience. Further, any activism either explicit or implicit by an individual shows how an equity in the balance of power this has been achieved by praxis.

## Feminism as identity ontology

In the historical reviews of literature above surrounding health psychology, identity, and feminism, the dualisms of mind/body, realism/

relativism, quantity/quality, oppressor/oppressed, determinism/agency and ideology/materialism are constant reminders of the issues of concern in these subjects. Based in Cartesian thinking, these dualisms have been shown to have progressed to more integrated theory based on the ontological subject and an epistemology aimed towards gathering knowledge based on a hermeneutic understanding of experience. This is an example of the generative process or synthesis between thesis and antithesis as well as progress from theory into praxis, which serves further to dissolve the dualisms, in health through the concept of embodiment of health identity in the experience of and action on the material world.

Dialectical thinking allows for the acknowledgement of these dualisms expressed as opposites on axes of power, but includes a relative aspect in that, because of the historical material nature of human experience each person's experience will, according to their unique historical psychosociocultural perspective differ from another person's perspective. People's perspectives will also vary due to the interaction of their relationship with the intransient effects of the natural world such as certain determined physical aspects and the natural world outside human control. These power relations, it must be noted, are not necessarily negative, but can also empower, as illustrated by the dialectics of illness and well-being in health psychology (Foucault, 1978). In the light of developments in theory and methodology, a review of the literature has highlighted the narrow nature of the study of the menopause and the perimenopause and consequently the ontological synthesis of health identity. From around 1980 there has been as advancement in critical philosophy, gendered health, feminist theory, health psychology in contrast to the halting of advancement created by continuing biomedical research into menopause and perimenopause. Advances in thinking and study have moved towards an integrated account of identity construction, taking and combining realist and relativist concepts into critical realism and the feminist standpoint. However, the study of women's health experience pertaining to the menopause and perimenopause has experienced a hiatus in thinking hampered by medical, political and economic concerns surrounding HRT and focusing on dualistic thinking.

For perimenopausal women, the social construction of their health identity has been inevitably centred around physical milestones such as menstruation, childbirth and the menopause, defined as 'sex' by the intransient natural world outside the control of humans. Gender, on the other hand, as a cultural construction in addition to a social construction, is more fluid and is defined by cultural expectation and stereotyping grounded in women as the 'weaker sex' and mediated as objectified. Illness and wellbeing in women, again often expressed and defined through physical milestones, are presented as the forefront in women's health through medical issues such as the physical symptoms of the menopause as defining factors and HRT as a cure all (Gannon & Stevens, 1998). But these natural watersheds in a woman's life are not discrete events, separate from other health concerns and vicariously experienced effects on identity. Past research has shown that ill health can cause serious identity disruption (Frank, 2000a). So how do women cope and strategise for health and wellbeing when faced with an inevitable event in their lives, such as the menopause, steeped in negative concepts (Rostosky & Travis, 1996) and looming large in their lives? In turn, and considering the interactive nature of identity construction, how do women incorporate non sex and gender specific illness and wellbeing and vicariously experienced representations and experiences of health and wellbeing into this feminised model of women's health?

## Societal discourses as competing ontology?

Society provides many discourses of women's health and identity. Gergen (1991) suggests that the impact of institutions in society such as religion, the media, medical organisations and the family all vie for a chance to influence people. The politics that impact upon women, health and feminism are competing with a patriarchal oriented society and the resulting discourses are charged with power dynamics. Gergen theorises this effect as saturation that competes for a place in the formation of identity.

Globalisation, which defines the world as becoming unitary in terms of economics, culture and politics, also impacts on the saturation of individuals by social discourses. Giddens (1998) describes globalisation as a situation where multiple discourses available on a world scale are available at one time which:

> ...generate a diversity of possible futures. (Giddens, 1998, p.5)

Gergen argues that as time goes on and technology increases, an ever-globalised society will lead to the increased saturation of the individual by diverse discourses all claiming to be 'truth'. As more discourses saturate society, more political opportunities to compete using power dynamics present themselves and the knowledge generation brought about by this competition to secure ontological status. An example of this is the competition within the HRT debate for ontological truth. Societal institutions such as medical organisation, the media, the government and the beauty industry have all been key players in the political battle to persuade women to take HRT. The campaigners for 'safe HRT' and the 'hormone rich and happy' women compete with those who wish to point out that HRT is risky. This political struggle has overarching competing ontological aspects such as capitalist ideals and feminist theory that reinforce the philosophical aspects of the struggle for the 'truth' about HRT. Women who are considering taking HRT will act on some of the discourses they interact with and ignore others depending on the level of information they receive.

Consequently, the heavier the saturation, the more reinforced the information becomes, and in the case of health, if action is taken on this information, it may become identity ontology.

## What do these competing ontologies mean for women's health identity?

We arrive here at a position where there are a number of competing ontologies available for a woman when constructing her health identity. Health information from the medical model of health provides an objectified version of the body typified by the listing of symptoms and the lack of any emotive material. Feminist epistemology focuses on a resistance to objectification of the female body. Societal discourses such as the media transmit the message of both and add its own construction of health in order to entice its audience, leaning towards objectification of the woman's body (Conboy et al., 1997). As a result of this, the lived health experience for women becomes confusing and dialectical. A constant issue involved in health choices, when faced with these competing discourses is the matter of truth. How does one decide which is true and therefore what to act on and embody in the world?

### Truth, power and knowledge: The impact of external constructions on women's health identity

So, identity construction is fluid and relational. Whilst an individual has choices in the way the information and knowledge received from personal, interpersonal, positional and situational (Murray, 2000) representations and discourses in society are constructed in their identity, these must first be made available in society as ontological objects and as 'truth'.

An example of 'truths' available to women in constructing their health identity as argued above are the medical model of health, feminist praxis and societal representations of health. However, at any one time, these discourses can all seem like the 'truth' because of the power dynamics involved in transmitting knowledge to the individual. Various aspects of society such as the concept of health itself, market forces and the environment all play a part in shaping the power dynamics between and amongst these discourses, all of which carry knowledge concerning health information along the whole of the dialectic from wellbeing to illness.

Identity construction often happens most forcefully when identity is in crisis. Information gathering and knowledge construction happens for a reason, and illness or the risk of illness is often a reason to find new information to make sense of illness or perceived risk of illness. Conversely, information about wellbeing is often not sought after as avidly as if a person does not have a problem with health and feels well, there is no crisis. This means that the information transmission needs to be more forceful to reach to audience i.e. the recipient of women's health information. The media, for example, is a main communicator of health information (O'Sullivan et al., 1994) and as a consequence is often made as attractive as possible to appeal to the drama and crisis that people require from interaction with the media (Maslow, 1968).

It is this power that constructs the various information as truth. Although much of the information is contradictory, it is often presented in society as a grand narrative of health through rhetoric of expertise (Bolam et al., 2003). From this grand narrative, women are able to construct the realities of their health identities.

## Truth and consumer politics

At first glance it would seem that there is no hope for women's health identity because of economic and political forces behind the various discourses of health (Marks et al., 2001) and the societal saturation of these impacting on women's health identity. Indeed, information concerning health seems overwhelming and oppressive in itself (Gergen, 1991). To some extent this is accurate, but this does not explain how, in the face of the potential for gaining knowledge about illness and wellbeing, some women continue to partake in risky health practices such as smoking and consumption of alcohol. If the power dynamic is so overwhelmingly oppressive in a hierarchical manner, why do women choose to ignore it?

The movement in social theory from modernity to postmodernism indicates the acknowledgement of the individual as re-theorised from the objective position of passive object in a 'cause and effect' model of determined identification to the subjective position of a person with a choice in the consumption societal discourses in a globalised, saturated world. This illustrates that people view information they are presented with and decide what the truth is. When there are conflicting 'truths', as there are in discourses of health, people are at liberty to switch from one 'truth' to another at will, and depending on the context and circumstances. This has an impact on identity construction, as identity as performed in one role may take up one health truth. For example, mothers may not smoke around their children, as they believe it will harm them, and this fits with the woman's 'nurturing' identity. In a social role with friends, the same woman may smoke outside a restaurant, fitting with an identity of camaraderie and social acceptance. Just as identity construction is relational, fluid and flexible, consumer representations in society are relative to each others power dynamics and economic forces. The media in its role as mediator of consumer politics is at will to change its story in order to sell itself and the product it is sponsored by – one week red wine is bad for your health as it will lead to alcoholism and the next week it is good for health as it lowers blood pressure. It would seem then, that just as identity is fluid, so is the representation of health 'truth'.

## Foucault and truth

The premise of a single truth suggests that those in possession of power are in possession of an absolute truth. However, as pointed out above, power dynamics involves a combination of economically and poliically fuelled discourses of what are often dialectical opposites. Foucault (1978) provides a philosophical explanation for this ever-changing model of society, identity and truth. Foucault rejects any absolute truth and provides a perspective from which to evaluate claims of truth.

Foucault's position on truth is not a theory as such, but more of a postmodern abstraction from which to view the discourses around which meaning is made. His work is based on the premise that in terms of history there is only fiction, because any recounting of history in discourse is a social construction. Consequently, there is no absolute or fixed reality, because from moment to moment the present becomes history. This means that there is no one fixed truth or reality in society; therefore, there can be no fixed theory that explains something. Taking this a step further, if theory or truth is not fixed and is fluid, power must also be fluid and open to change depending on the relation variation in society such as changing political views and the economy. For example, some theorists (Chomsky, 1989; Marx, 1954; Weber, 1962) believe that power is dependant on hierarchical domination by many privileged groups who will oppress and will stay oppressors as long as they are privileged. Foucault, however, comments that power is not unitary and is not absolute. He suggests that power is dispersed in society relationally through discourse. Foucault does not suggest that the power struggle is not unequal, but intimates that it is not just directed in a single downward spiral.

The concept of freedom is important to Foucault's works, as he maintains that without it there can be no power; power on dialectic can only have an effect if the object of the power is able to recognise it and resist. The power of the patriarchal model of health and feminist theories' resistance to the objectified woman's body in health is an example of this.

Enlarging on Foucault's view that history is fiction and the present is not reality because of the fleeting nature of the moment into history, the application of knowledge to the present is also relational and fictional. Therefore, on a personal level, the application of any knowledge will only create a perceived truth that is not reality. However, this perceived truth will still be represented in the identity, however fleetingly, and in meaning-making may influence action. In this context, it is reasonable to assume that more than one perceived truth can be taken from society, even contradictory perceived truths, and be actioned according to social context including the media.

## Critical realism, truth and the lived experience

The lived experience of women today inevitably involves some contact with politics, with health concepts and with concepts of equality. Women are concerned about their health and the focus of women's health is around the reproductive cycle and the milestones in this cycle such as puberty, menstruation, childbirth and the menopause. Whilst postmodernism provides multiple positions to observe the identity construction of women in a fluid and relational way, it is congruent with the social and ideal realms of Bhaskar's empirical domain of perceived experience, and goes some way to contribute to an explanation of the general mechanisms of truth, power and knowledge, a vital part of lived experience is missed.

Critical realist thinking provides a model that allows for the important reality of the corporeal body (in Bhaskar's actual domain) and for the fact that whatever we will allow the body to do, it continues with the reproductive cycle until death. This is not to say that intervention cannot change some part of the reproductive cycle, for example sterilisation or hysterectomy, but to suggest that this removes the reproductive cycle completely due to loss of fertility would be to resort to Cartesian thinking of 'woman as womb'. In fact, the whole endocrine system is involved in reproduction, and even when the womb is removed, the pituitary gland still produces lutenising hormones.

Critical realist thinking, rather than taking the furthest point on the dialectical axis of the realist/relativist debate, lies near the middle of the axis, depending on the circumstances of the situation. In the human situation, and particularly concerning health, where the corporeal body cannot be ignored, critical realism takes into account the positivist scientific health paradigm pertaining to the actual domain but also acknowledges the holistic model of health psychology that includes the inevitable feelings and emotions concerning the health condition. This is combined into an interactive model of the actual, the empirical and the real domains which considers the corporeal body and its illness/wellbeing, the social construction of feelings around health and the mechanisms which draw the two together, which are relative and postmodern in nature.

This critique of the realist and positivist position requires acknowledgement of the values of empirical work. It does not hold these as truths but as relational realities that, whilst they cannot be discounted, are one of several differing discourses of health. This allows for a qualitative holistic study of material and socially constructed aspects of the lived health experience, taking into account feelings and emotions concerning the health situation, whilst paying attention to the perceived pathology of the corporeal body and the meaning-making around wellbeing and body.

## Critical realism, postmodernism, reflexivity and narrative psychology: Historical fiction?

The discussion above has focused on critical realist and postmodern perspectives of epistemology, ontology and truth in terms of relative power and knowledge constructions of competing discourses in society. These discourses are presented in the form of theory transmitted in society and available as competing truths. Consequently, individuals choose which discourses to internalise, depending on their unique social, political and economic position and situation. Also present are theories of identity to explain how people perform their identity in society and these are transmitted to society through academic studies, including health identity. As discussed previously, much of health identity theorisation has been produced through a positivist medical model of health.

This interaction of powerful discourses in society competing for positions of truth and the restrictions of the medical model of health in terms of realist and positivist methodology has excluded the exploration of health identity from a person-centred standpoint (Rogers, 1951). Additionally, patriarchal hegemonic influences on society have objectified women's bodies, negating the need to investigate the feelings and emotions involved in women's health. As a result of this, women's voices in health research are rarely heard. That is not to say that women who do research are in the minority. Women who train in positivist and empirical scientific methodology and use this to carry out health research are suffering a form of censorship through the institutional patriarchy in which they are based, for example, the medical model of health based in hypothesis driven statistical work and regulation of scientific presentation of papers. This 'feminist as far as possible' position is similar to Beauvoir's 'independent woman' (De Beauvoir, 1949) who provides her own income only to submit to patriarchy and hegemony by asserting her independence by conforming to media dictated fashion.

Social scientists are now taking up the challenge of critical health psychology in order to investigate the qualitative health dynamics that the quantitative medical model of health has largely ignored. The feelings, attitudes and emotions of women in women's health psychology have been difficult to examine because of the focus on the objectified reproductive cycle of the corporeal body. The patriarchal view of 'woman as womb' that pervades society has overpowered the need for women to explain subjectively how their health is affected by different issues. The normalisation of women through various societal grand narratives and discourses has reinforced the ideology of objectification, and may leave women confused when they become unhappy with, or do not fit into a prescribed category or trend; this dissatisfaction has contributed to the rise of feminist thinking.

For the working class woman in Oldham, who has had little opportunity to publicly question the medical model of health or the social construction of women, the saturation of the powerful and competitive discourses of society may be oppressive. How can these women be empowered and have their voices heard above the white noise of positivist study, where they will inevitably be made invisible as a number?

## Theory to praxis through the narrative account

Critical realist thinking suggests the necessity of using qualitative research to explore the human situation because of the double hermeneutic (Ginev, 1998). The double hermeneutic is the concept of understanding on both sides of the research. In positivist research, subjective understanding occurs only on the side of the researcher; the research object is passive. The double hermeneutic recognises the active mutable subject in both the researcher and the subject under research. The phenomenon of people studying people is inherently subjective and interpretive; in order to study the relational lived experience and identity, it is necessary to take into account the complex interrelationship between individual and society. However, in accepting this position it is also necessary to be mindful that, if multiple and shifting truths or ontologies are possible in society, and identity construction is fluid and changing, then what an individual perceives as the truth is relative.

Identity epistemology and ontology, whilst socially constructed, will be perceived as the truth by the individual until such time as the identity is in crisis and this truth is questioned. The performance of the historical individual health identity through a narrative lifespan account, then, can be studied by obtaining an autobiographical storied account of lived health experience. This will clarify how a woman perceives embodied health and how this has changed over time and is perceived for the future. Additionally, incongruencies in society such as political issues and social injustice will be exposed in relation to the lived experience of the women who take part in this study. As Giddens (1991) points out:

> The self today is a reflexive project – a more or less continuous interrogation of past, present and future. It is a project carried on amid a profusion of reflexive resources; therapy and self help manuals of all kinds, television programmes and magazine articles. (Giddens, 1991, p.30)

The critical realist approach taken here allows for a postmodernist relativist investigation of the complex interaction of society and identity whilst acknowledging the importance of the corporeal body and the meaning-making properties of individuals in illness and wellbeing.

Ricoeur (1983) argues that the telling of the narrative story and the construction of the autobiography is the transmission of the identity into praxis, when one becomes responsible for the meaning-making reflexive account of how we perceive our lives to be. Caution must be taken in the assumption that an individual creates meaning in an agentic way, because, as we have seen, many complex and tacit power dynamics are involved in the relational identity construction and these may not be made explicit in the retelling of the narrative.

It is this factor that makes the autobiographical narrative account a useful methodological tool for the investigation of women's health identity. Contained in the information-rich narrative accounts of the lived experience (Crossley, 2000b; Frank, 2000a; McAdams, 1993; Mishler, 1999) are metaphors of power dynamics and imagery, which link the personal narrative to experiences on an interpersonal, positional and situational level in society. The way in which the story is told is also important as this also shows the pervading tone of the narrative due to the historically situated position. Through studying narrative accounts of perimenopausal women, who have experiences of many physiological milestones of the corporeal body, the meaning-making around these milestones will be explored and how they have been embodied in experience. By analysing the narrative accounts on the levels of the personal, the interpersonal and the institutional (Murray, 2000) aspects of identity in terms of themes, images and tones (Crossley, 2000b; McAdams, 1993), the construction of women's health identity in terms of explicitly stated personal and vicariously experienced health constructions and the less transparent issues of power dynamics in society that affect health will be explored.

To recap, in order to investigate a critical person-centred approach to the investigation of perimenopausal health and identity construction:

- a critical approach to health in order to include social, economic, cultural and political aspects of health in addition to personal health can be taken
- women's gendered health and identity using this critical approach can be assessed
- a postmodern notion of fluid and fragmented health identity can be used as a model
- feminist standpoint theory, underpinned by a critical realist philosophical approach is appropriate

- methodology capable of investigating health identity construction in terms of the above points to collect data from the participants in the study using a critical approach such as narrative psychology will be used

In the following chapters, an autobiographical account of the construction of health identity amongst perimenopausal women in the light of a critical approach and following the points above will be given as evidence of the multi-level, multi-domain nature of identity construction.

# 5 Investigating Women's Health: The Story So Far

## Introduction

This chapter, which connects theory of health and identity with investigation of health and identity, provides a stepping-stone between concept and people. The central aim is to investigate the individual experiences of women aged between 35–55 in relation to how their health identity is constructed and embodied throughout their life and to find out the impact of societal issues on these experiences. In addition to this, the study is grounded in a critical approach that considers social, cultural and political aspects of experience. In order to investigate how perimenopausal women construct their health identity and locate narratives within society, the following question, which has been considered in the theory chapters, is still pertinent to address these issues:

*What health considerations have perimenopausal women undergone in lived experience and how have they used these to construct a health identity?*

The approach, design and method of this qualitative study, is explained in this chapter so that this study can be replicated, re-analysed or at least applied to other questions of understanding social change.

## Why use qualitative methodology?

The research methodology is qualitative throughout this project as the aim are to investigate the lived experience of the women by examining their account of feelings, emotions and attitudes in relation to their health and how these contribute to their health identity. This is so that the women involved are given a voice through which they can express their lived experience in the context of health identity and this can be heard through the study, not hidden behind quantified generalisation.

A rigorous adherence to validity and replicable testing and analysis on the basis of statistics and generalisation in quantitative methodology do not attend to the complexity and fluidity of the rich lived experience. The aim of qualitative methodology is for the researcher to study an issue or problem and interpret the issue or problem through reflexive contemplation.

Whilst quantitative methodology aims to eliminate subjectivity in favour of objectivity in order to obtain validity, reliability and generalisation, qualitative methodology embraces subjectivity and interpretation as flexible and fluid. Moreover, Ratner (2002) comments that:

> Qualitative methodology recognises that the subjectivity of the researcher is intimately involved in scientific research. Subjectivity guides everything from the choice of topic that one studies, to formulating hypotheses, to selecting methodologies, and interpreting data. In qualitative methodology, the researcher is encouraged to reflect on the values and objectives he brings to the research project. Other researchers are also encouraged to reflect on the values that any particular investigator utilizes. (Ratner, 2002)

This is not to say that qualitative research is not valid and reliable. However, these terms are reframed in qualitative research in terms of authenticity and interpretation.

### Authenticity and interpretation in qualitative research

Whereas validity in quantitative research is concerned with controlling the variables under research to extract certain information, qualitative research tries to ensure authenticity by including as many situations as possible to make the research setting a holistic part of the person's lived experience. Reliability in quantitative research ensures the measurement used in the research is replicable whereas reliability in qualitative research:

> Has more to do with reinterpreting the findings from a different standpoint or exploring the same issues in different contexts. (Banister et al., 1998, p.143)

Generalisability is also problematic for qualitative research, particularly critical psychology. In positivist-quantified research, great efforts are made to produce generalisable results that may predict some aspect of human behaviour of society. However, a critical approach aims not at a result in terms of absolute findings, but of an understanding of the dynamics of the matter under investigation. The interpretation and reinterpretation of findings from critically designed studies is more important than results which are one-dimensional and quantified (Sapsford, 1987).

The problem of objectification and objectivity in research when studying people and their feelings, emotions and attitudes extends to the subject of reflexivity. In this project, the subjectivity of the women interviewed was respected and interpreted their accounts accordingly. In line with qualitative work aims, it is aimed to make the study as authentic as possible by including varied lived experiences in the study. Narrative psychology, as discussed in the previous chapter, is an available qualitative methodology that allows for a critical approach to health research.

## What is narrative psychology?

Narrative psychology is a methodology that is concerned with the 'storied nature of human conduct' and aims to explain how people construct and reconstruct experience by narrating stories and listening to the stories of others (Sarbin, 1986). It provides a way of studying the self that takes into account linguistic, historical and social structures (Crossley, 2000b). It allows researchers to examine the connection between how people explain the way that they live and how they experience the self in the context of social, moral, cultural and political aspects of society. It also relies on language as a tool for constructing reality. Researchers studying narratives are challenged by the theory that human activity and experience are filled with meaning and that stories are the vehicle by which that meaning is communicated as opposed to the logical arguments or lawful formulations of more structured approaches (Andrews et al., 2008).

### Why use narrative psychology?

Narrative methodology was chosen for this project as it provides an opportunity to study a whole life autobiographical account of lived experience. This is important when investigating considerations of health as the health identity is cumulative and is a whole life construction, taking into account all aspects of women's health. Additionally, narrative psychology methodology provides an opportunity to investigate, through these autobiographical accounts, the personal, interpersonal and societal power dynamics related to health that are experienced by the women who took part in this study. As the research field is a deprived economic area in the North of England, this important context of the study contributes to the lived health experience. The aims are to deconstruct the autobiographical accounts of the participants and identify personal, interpersonal and societal aspects of the accounts so as to argue for a fragmented but interactive construction of health identity and narrative methodology which will assist in this.

This methodology was also selected for use in this study due to the explanatory nature of the narrative approach. (Crossley, 2000b; McAdams, 1993; Mishler, 1995). Frank (2000a) defends narrative analysis from various criticisms of quantitatively oriented psychology by pointing out that the relationship between the researcher and participant:

> A social scientist who engages the story shares this problem of how to sustain his or her part in the network of relationships created by the story. (Frank, 2000a, p.355)

The observation of narrative methodology points out the need to embed the lived experience in the social world, noting social and cultural levels of analysis alongside the personal and interpersonal. Whilst this is true of discourse analysis and qualitative work in general, narrative analysis brings a more personal perspective by considering the temporal emplotment of the whole life story and examining the personal account in addition to the discourses within the account. This in turn allows for a person-centred account to emerge, which empowers the subject and not the discourse (Rogers, 1951). Mishler (1995) goes on to explain about narrative form and the construction of the story with a temporal order and structure; a beginning, a succession of happenings and an end. Mishler justifies the story over a set of instructions by stating that these stories have 'causality, implicativeness or thematic order' (Mishler, 1995). Steps carried out in sequence as in the form of a set of instructions are different from stories in an important way: meaning.

### Narratives and identity

Meaning is the ingredient that ties the telling of the story with the identity. The historically temporal aspects of the narrative concur with Foucauldian discourse analysis and the genealogical or historical timeline methodology employed (Foucault, 1978). Similarly, the discourse/power/knowledge triad is implicated in narrative study within the inherent social and cultural involvement in the storied identity.

Roberts (2003) examines the construction of identity through narrative and comments that in telling our stories:

> The unceasing quest is to give an understanding and form to experience, to locate us in place and time, to situate ourselves in webs of relations. (Roberts, 2003, p.121)

In explaining their life in everyday terms, people tell stories to bring order, continuity and coherence to their experiences (Roberts, 2003). The role of the narrative researcher, according to Roberts, is to bring this storytelling into the research area as realistically as possible. Roberts stresses that although the concept of time is important in the narrative, the timeline of the narrative may not always run in chronological order, particularly in more chaotic narratives. To address this potential problem for narrative researchers McAdams (1993) developed a method to investigate the cumulative identity in a more structured way. By requesting that the story is told according to life chapters, the participant is encouraged to think of their experiences in terms of a structured story. Crossley (2000b) has developed this method and comments that:

> Everything experienced by human beings is made meaningful, understood and interpreted in relation to the primary dimension of 'activity': this incorporated both 'time' and 'sequence'. (Crossley, 2000b, p.10)

and also stresses that personal relationships are important when constructing meaning in identity:

> When we ask ourselves the question 'what does this mean?' we are asking ourselves (or others) *how* something is related or connected to something or someone else. (Crossley, 2000b, p.11)

This method of designing the study according to the structures of time and relationships produces a chronological linear account of the lived experience through which identity construction in terms of meaning can be studied.

In constructing the narrative from memory, important events which happen in lived experience, are brought into the story in order to give a coherent meaning to the story (Collins and Nicolson, 2002). These peak and nadir experiences (McAdams, 1993) signal peaks and troughs in the narrative that imply points in the lived experience which are meaningful in terms of the issues which occur in the construction of identity. McAdams (1993) examines these 'narrative disjoins' in terms of the personal narrative and Frank (2000a) extends this to the health narrative to illustrate these disjoins, and how they affect specific aspects of identity construction, in this case, health identity. In the context of health identity construction, disjoins in the narrative account, which can be either peak or nadir experiences, provide a particular clear and strong point in the story where change is marked. In terms of this book, use of narrative psychology will attempt to expose the health stories of the women who take part in an ordered fashion to allow for deconstruction into different levels of analysis. However, because of the multidirectional timeline of the narrative account and the narrative disjoins as explained above, it will be possible to locate the women's health identity construction in the story in a chronological nature in addition to identifying identity in times of crisis and change in the context of health.

## Women's narratives

The narrative psychology methodology used in this investigation is aptly applied to qualitative enquiry into women's health. Narrative methodology does not specifically take into account gender differences although this gap is partially filled by McAdams (1993) in the explanation of how relationship narratives highlight the emotional differences in gender. The general health identity of women is not cited as a reason for narrative disjoins from a feminist perspective in these texts.

However, by incorporating the postmodern feminist thinking of difference within difference, as discussed in Chapter 3, the life story can be studied as an isolated non-comparative event. The narrative focuses on the participant as a contributor to the research and owner of their story (Crossley, 2000b), diffusing the gender-centred power relationship with the implicitly reflexive position of the researcher in the retelling of the story in analysis (Mishler, 1995). In terms of health identity, accounts of women's health have previously been embedded in a medicalised model. By using narrative methodology, accounts of women's health are lifted from the medicalised model and placed in a more person-centred context. This exposes the women's accounts of the experiences a medicalised model imposing on their experience within the sub-narratives disjoins of the health experience. These are typically storied through an interaction of social, cultural and political explanations.

A feminist approach and narrative methodology is therefore appropriate to study identity construction in women's health. However, whilst the collection of data using narrative methodology provides information rich storied accounts of the lived experience, the task of analysis is of equal importance when representing women's voices.

## Narrative methodology and analysis

With the resurgence of narrative psychology methodology in recent years, because of its suitability and ease of application to critical approaches, there are many ways to do narrative research. Data collection, in the form of the narrative account, can be conducted using varying degrees of structure in the interview schedule, ranging from a single question eliciting a free-narrative story to a list of strictly imposed interview questions eliciting a guided story.

Similarly, and connected to data collection and the aims of this particular study, several different models of narrative analysis are available. As the aim of narrative analysis is to investigate how the world is storied and how these stories make meaning, the aims of the study and the specific research question are extremely pertinent to the type of narrative analysis used. Narrative methods widely vary from free flowing, unstructured and abstract interpretations of the outcomes of the study to structured reporting on aspects under investigation.

## Levels of analysis

The approach used in the study is based on McAdams (1993) model of narrative enquiry which is designed to draw out the historical sequence of life events. By asking specific questions about peak experience and nadir experience, important people and the formation of life chapter, life themes and future expectations, McAdams aims to investigate the emotive past of a person and how the sequence of socio-cultural input has shaped the themes of a life and the expectations for the future. Mishler's (1999) contribution of the concept of the disjoined narrative investigated how personal milestones (negative or positive) can serve as identity intervention and markers for change. This model of narrative psychology allows for external influences and experiences to be accounted for in the narrative. Expanding on this concept, Murray's (2000) paper examines how the subjective experiential nature of narrative accounts can be expanded to a multi-level analysis in line with a model of health psychology that encompasses the biological, social, and cultural in interaction with psychological aspects of health. Murray considers the character of health and illness narratives as a function of the personal, interpersonal, positional and societal levels of analysis (Murray, 2000):

> At the personal level of analysis narratives are portrayed as expressions of the lived experience of the narrator. At the interpersonal level of analysis the narrative is one that is co-created in conversation (i.e. in the interview). At the positional level of analysis the analysis considers the differences in social position between the narrator and the listener. The societal level of analysis is concerned with the socially shared stories that are characteristic of certain communities or societies. (Murray, 2000, p.337)

This expansion of the narrative account further enhances the use of this approach in critical health psychology by including the psycho-socio-cultural functions of the personal narrative. Contributions on the societal level of the narrative often come from the external world in the form of representations from society such as family, media, medical and gendered discourses.

Additionally, a comparative aspect of narrative study can be used to compare and contrast the socially constructed health identity through the thematic analysis of the narrative accounts. It is the concept of the investigation of the in-depth individual's lived experience of health as a starting point that underpins the narrative approach taken in this study.

## How the work was carried out

This study used narrative methods and in order to collect data individual interviews with the women who participated in the study were carried out. The first step in this was to identify the sample. In order to recruit women for this study an advertisement was placed in a local newspaper and a poster placed in various locations around the study site. The response to this advert was high, with 247 telephone responses offering participation. Sixty three of the potential participants turned out to be outside the age range for the study, and 184 women within the age range were sent a participant pack. Twenty-seven women returned the participant pack and attended an informal meeting where they completed the participant pack, agreeing to commit to the study.

The aim of the study was to investigate the lived experience and identity construction of perimenopausal women, and how this is located in society. The sample generated therefore needed to include a targeted sample of women between the ages of 35–55 as this is deemed to be the perimenopausal transition period (Samisoe, 2002).

Thirty-two participants in total took part in this study and all the interviews were conducted individually with the participant. Each participant was interviewed twice as appropriate or wherever possible. The first interview included a general health lifespan request designed to draw out a story of health including past, present and future expectations. The second interview questions were designed to draw out any peak and nadir experiences in addition to any important relationships that may influence health identity (Crossley, 2000b). Fifteen participants agreed to be interviewed a second time. Seventeen participants either declined a second interview or could not be contacted. All the women who declined a second interview spoke of how they felt they had exhausted their health stories in the first interview. All the interviews were recorded on a tape recorder and a selection of them transcribed including 20 first interviews and five second interviews. The interviews transcribed were those, which, on listening to the tapes, contained the most information rich material and most relevant to this study. The remainder were closely studied and detailed notes were made. An interview summary was made after each meeting to incorporate any important themes and comments that were made by the women. Following this the interviews were analysed according to the narrative methods as described earlier in this chapter.

## Interviewing women

What makes feminist research 'feminist' is a challenge to the scientism that refuses to address the relations between knowledge (and knowledge-generating practices) and power, and a corresponding attention to reflexive issues in the form of theorizing and transforming the process of academic production, including the position of the researcher (Banister et al., 1998, p.123). Whilst not all qualitative study involves interviewing women, the feminist approach to interviewing provides a pertinent model to explain power imbalance in interviews and its aptness to this study.

Oakley (1981) notes that the interview, whilst being a form of conversation, is also a method of collecting data. The interview must work within the boundaries of the focus of the study to collect the data needed. Additionally, the study must be designed to ask the questions to which answers would be relevant to the area of study. Whereas quantitative study would isolate the focal issue and control it as a variable, qualitative study is inclusive of meaning-making surrounding interactions of lived experience. Consequently, in initiating qualitative research, the researcher imbues the process with his or her own thoughts, feelings and emotions regarding the focal issue. In designing the study, the reflexive researcher designs an inquiry using a methodology, which aims to explore a holistic account of how the participant lives in the context of the research questions. In order to obtain the account of the participant the study design must involve some kind of personal interaction between the researcher and the participant. One method often used to obtain such personal accounts, and the method used in this study, is the interview.

However, implicit in this consideration is the pre-conceived notion of both the researcher and the participant of what the interview actually is. Oakley (1981) explains that the interview emerged out of positivist science and is generally regarded as a male activity. The dynamic implicated in interviewing is that the interviewer is in a more powerful position due to status and knowledge directly related to the elevated status of interviewer. Feminist theory has contested this dynamic and attempted to equate the power dynamic by designing the study so that by conducting the interview, the research is empowering the interviewee. However, Tang (2002) argues that:

> Both the interviewers and the interviewees perceptions of social, cultural and personal differences have the impact on power relationships in the interview, which is not simply an issue of quality of the interview, but the dynamics between the interview pair. (Tang, 2002, p.703)

Luff (1999) comments that:

> ...it is helpful to think of 'moments of rapport' within the interview context, and to explore these moments as potentially rich sources of insight, theoretically and methodologically. An awareness of and attention to specific moments of rapport, as well of moments of disjuncture, in woman to woman interviews seems crucial if feminist researchers are to acknowledge differences and divisions between women. (Luff, 1999, p.701)

Luff's work on feminist research with non-feminist women highlights the potential difficulties of being unable to know the participants' position on personal, social and cultural issues prior to the research. On the same subject, Kim (1997) adds that the process of traditional research maintains rather than diffuses traditional power relationships in research. This brings into question the possibility of ever being able to diffuse the power dynamic in feminist research. However, this point is addressed to some extent by the explicit inclusion of the reflexive position of the researcher during qualitative research and the acknowledgement of awareness of this position during the study design, the collection of personal accounts from the participant and the analysis.

Many feminist researchers have used autobiographical narrative methods such as interviews to obtain accounts of the lived experience due to the open-ended structure of the life story and the opportunity this gives to explore issues of power. Narrative psychology provides a backdrop for these methods.

### Semi-structured interviews

The interview is a widely used method of collecting narrative accounts (Mishler, 1999) and the semi-structured interview was used to collect narrative data in this study. Interview protocol can take many forms, from a set list of interview questions, to a completely open-ended interview with no set questions. The semi-structured interview is useful in narrative methodology as Crossley (2000b) explains:

> ...a 'semi-structured' interview which basically means that the list of questions set out in the protocol serve as a guide rather than something that should be strictly adhered to. (Crossley, 2000b, p.267)

Oakley (1981) highlighted the problematic nature of interviewing women due to power dynamics and the hierarchical status of the interviewer–interviewee relationship. Oakley comments that:

> ...it becomes clear that, in most cases, the goal of finding out about people through interviewing is best achieved when the relationship of interviewer and interviewee is non-hierarchical and when the interviewer is prepared to invest his or her own personal identity in the relationship. (Oakley, 1981, p.273)

Feminist narrative interviewing, then, requires that the researcher, armed with a set of questions, conduct an interview with as few power dynamics as possible. To accommodate this, semi-structured interviews are conducted on a fairly open framework using the interview schedule as a guideline for introduction of topic, and introducing further appropriate questions as the interview progresses. Larson (1997) examined the narrative inquiry process and concluded that to achieve a rapport a dialogue must take place between the researcher and participant. This dialogue is not simply the asking of a particular question, to be answered by the participant, but the injection of empathetic input into the research conversation itself. Otherwise:

> By failing to engage in deliberative dialogue and inquiry, researchers put themselves at greater risk of not seeing, not understanding, and misinterpreting people whose lives and life experiences differ from their own. (Larson, 1997, p.459)

By using a semi-structured interview the researcher is guided by the main issues of the research but free to interject into the interview at any point with pertinent dialogue.

The semi-structured interviews in this study were constructed using a set of health-related questions that were applied in the interviews. This set of questions was intended as a guide to the interview and the questions were left open-ended so that the participants felt that they were able to express their own account of their health life.

### The interview schedule

The questions included in the interview schedule were based on a narrative approach (Crossley, 2000b; McAdams, 1993) that was intended to draw out life experience across the lifespan. The first item on the interview schedule, which is more of a request than a question and which is addressed in the first interview, asks that experiences of health be divided into 'life chapters'. The aim was to provide the participant with a type of storyboard framework, which assists both the researcher and the participant to form a coherent basis for organisation of the narrative account.

The second and subsequent questions, which are addressed in the second interview, cover peak and nadir experiences in different chronological stages of the participant's life.

The interviews were face to face and conducted at the homes of the participants' by previous appointment or by telephone. Where possible, a pre-interview meeting was arranged to explain the purpose of the study and the nature of the interview so as to diffuse the hierarchical power dynamics of the interview process (Christodoulou, 2006; Oakley, 1981). This helped both the researcher and the participant to become more familiar and to establish a relationship before the formal interview process began, and to resolve any questions or issues about the study.

**Data analysis of semi-structured interviews**

The semi-structured interview questions were used as a guideline during the interview conversation between the participant and researcher. The conversations were recorded on a tape recorder then transcribed the tape using a transcription machine. Care was taken to ensure that the accounts were rigorously transcribed as this adds to the validity of the research, according to Easton et al. (2000). Transcription and the care taken in repeated listening to the words and tones of the participant are an important part of the interpretation process, according to Easton et al. the same care was taken with those interviews that detailed notes were made on, the tapes of these interviews were listened to many times. Where the participant stated that they felt uncomfortable speaking into the microphone, contemporaneous notes were taken, and with the permission of the participant, were included in the study. The transcript was then subjected to analysis that investigated the tones, images and themes of the lived experience.

**Tones, themes and images**

The tone, themes and images of the interview was gauged by not only the textual content of the narrative but also the manner in which it was told (Crossley, 2000b). The tone of the interview is an important aspect of the analysis in that it provides a backdrop of understanding the main themes of the narrative. Images are important in the narrative account as they provide an explicit link from the personal experience to the interpersonal, positional and situational aspect of the narrative account (Murray, 2000). Themes are patterns that run through the narrative account and point to important overarching dynamics in the account. Themes that run through the narrative are often apparent at the beginning of the life chapters. Examples of themes that were explored in this study are women's health in terms of health milestones, such as menstruation and the perimenopause in addition to wellbeing, from the personal perspective of the health identity; relational experiences of women's health such as PMS and fertility from the interpersonal perspective of identity; also institutionalised health experiences such as medicalised health experiences and spirituality from the positional and ideological more implicitly experienced health in society.

## The research site

In order to take a critical approach to this study, the details of the situated health context of the women were considered in the area where they live. The women in this study were currently located in the North West of England and lived in Oldham, an economically challenged regeneration area. The health profile of this area was lower than the national level with more incidences of chronic diseases and disability. The number of people claiming welfare benefits in the area was high, as was the rate of teenage pregnancy and unemployment. Additionally, the number of single parent families was higher than the national average. In the context of health, a news headline in a local newspaper at the time of the study announced that 10 per cent of the borough are 'on the sick'. The article goes on to explain that more than one in ten of the research site's workforce was on long-term sickness benefits lasting six months or more. The annual consultation for public health details was cause for concern in the town in relation to challenging health inequalities in the research site (Public Health Report, 2004). The report recognised the risk factors of smoking, physical activity, healthy eating, alcohol and sexual health as predictors of the health of the area, which had several problem areas where predicted incidence of long term or terminal illness was often much higher than the national average and life expectancy consequently lower than the national average.

The report recognises serious health inequalities in the town and aims to address these through interventions such as promoting access to smoke free environments, uptake of health eating and uptake of physical activity. As previously mentioned in Chapter 1, the research site is positioned at 38$^{th}$ in the 'Indices of Deprivation', a measurement of deprivation in communities as constructed by the government.

## The participants

The participants were women aged 35–55 who expressed an interest in taking part in the research after seeing the poster or newspaper article appealing for interest. All the participants could be described as working class even though this was not a recruitment strategy. Thirty of the participants had lived in the Manchester area all of their lives and were white. Two of the participants were of second-generation Asian ethnic origin and had been born in Oldham. All the participants worked either as housewives or in outside employment. Twelve were married and out of these three were widowed. Eight of the women lived with a partner, five were single, and seven were divorced and 22 had children, eight had grandchildren. Eight of the participants considered themselves to have long-term health problems such as heart disease, arthritis or asthma. Two of the participants stated that they were gay during the interviews. The mean age of the participants was 46 years.

## Ethical considerations

At the outset of this study, ethical approval was granted and the interviews were conducted according to British Psychological Society Guidelines (re: BPS Guidelines, 2000). Care was taken to inform the participants through the participant pack and during the initial meeting of the ethical issues related to participation in the study. Each participant was informed of the nature of the study and how the data would be presented in the report or in presentations or in published material. The participant was reassured throughout the research as to the anonymity of the participant in the report (Banister et al., 1998) and informed consent acquired.

Informed consent, in this case, included a contract that was signed by the researcher and the participant. This detailed a paragraph about anonymity in the study that was also explained during the initial interviews. Care was taken to explain the difference between anonymity and confidentiality to the participants, as it emerged that that there might be some confusion between the two. Geertz (1973) cautions the use of anonymity in thick descriptive accounts and hence all the participants' names and personal details were changed in the narrative accounts.

## Chapter summary

This chapter has detailed the methodology, methods and procedures used to carry out this study. It has established that in order to study perimenopausal identity construction:

- A suitable sample for the study has been obtained
- A narrative methodology has been successfully applied and used for the individual interviews
- Ethical considerations have been observed
- Transcripts and notes of the interviews have been produced and analysed

In the following chapters the analysis of the autobiographical accounts in the context of the construction of women's health identity will be presented.

# Part II

# Voice

The previous theory section supports an idea of identity construction, in this case pertaining to women's health that is supported by a suitable theoretical, philosophical methodological framework.

Whilst theory provides a landscape for identity construction evidence is needed that what is argued for occurs in lived experience. The following section gives a voice to the often taken-for-granted, everyday occurrence of identity construction. Beginning from a personal perspective the voices grow louder as identity construct stretches through interpersonal relationships and into society.

The theory comes alive with the voices of 32 women who talk about their health and identity in rich narratives that express lived experience.

# 6
# Narrative Touchstones of the Storied Perimenopausal Health Identity

## Introduction

Whilst information about women's health saturates society through various representations (Lyons, 2000), the effect that these representations have on the formation of women's health identity construction remains largely unreported by the voices of the women themselves. This is reflected in the following question used to investigate this issue:

*What health considerations have perimenopausal women undergone in lived experience and how have they used these to construct a health identity?*

The aim of this study was to address this and investigate these health considerations by re-presenting the individual health experiences of women using the narratives of perimenopausal women from Oldham, a deprived community in Northern England. The following narratives will help to understand how lived experience contributes to considerations of health and how these help to construct health identity, in addition to what these health considerations mean to the women who took part in the study. In order to address these issues the women's accounts were deconstructed in terms of personal, interpersonal, ideological, and positional aspects of health identity (Murray, 2000). This allowed illustration the self-evaluation and monitoring of personal health in order to emphasise the way the participants construct their personal health identity through the plot of the account. Additionally, the interpersonal health experience can be examined through accounts of embodied health and reciprocal and integrated health experiences with other people, and the effects on these on the construction of health identity. Finally, the ideological and positional experience of health through institutionalised power dynamics in society is examined through exposing the participant's implicit experiences of the medical model of health, feminist health, media, family and spiritual discourses that affect health experiences. In this multilayered model of the construction and re-construction of the perimenopausal health identity, the analysis of tones, themes and images in the accounts provide insight into the rich depth of the storied lives of the participants (Crossley, 2000b; McAdams, 1993). The depth of these accounts reveals points of reference or touchstones of health used by the women to plot their health life story. This emplotment, which is one way women construct their health life stories, brings order to the chaotic nature of identity construction (Roberts, 2003). The socially constructed material milestones of women's health such as menstruation, pregnancy, childbirth and menopause are clearly present in the accounts. However, the experience of these and embodiment of material milestones may be touchstones of the way women live in terms of their health relationships with themselves, others and society.

## Stories of health

The narratives were divided between two types of sub-narrative story. These were stories that differed from each other in narrative style and were non-temporal. The first of these was the generic story of health that was presented as discreet events in the narrative account. This included stories about many different non-gender specific health problems that ranged from chronic problems such as varicose veins to terminal health problems such as heart failure and cancer.

The second sub-narrative was organised around women's reproductive health milestones and followed a pattern throughout the narrative in order of these milestones using them as narrative touchstones that linked the personal and the social. Whilst the narratives progressed temporally through the natural physiologically fixed milestones of menstruation, pregnancy, childbirth towards perimenopause, these were not the only temporal events which formed the basis of the women's health sub-narrative. Other medical interventions such as abortion, sterilisation and hysterectomy were also experienced as reproductive milestones of women's lives. In this study, the medical narrative of symptom listing and milestone listing resembled an ongoing set of components. It was the relational narrative that moved the story on and linked the narrative together in terms of temporal form, location, characters and plots that made the story of the construction of health identity, not solely isolated medical events.

Unlike the generic health stories, the women's reproductive health stories were mostly pathological in nature. None of the women talked about reproductive health in terms of wellbeing and when speaking about their periods used the words 'horrendous', 'painful' and 'disruptive'. Similarly, when discussing the menopause, words such as 'intrusive', 'groggy', 'dark' and 'downhill' were used. This suggests that, unlike the generic health stories, the women had no clear examples of personal or vicarious coping experiences to refer to in order to reframe their reproductive health and it may be that women's health is a more personalised experience. Further, medical interventions were often seen as the only option for wellbeing in reproductive health perhaps illustrating a lack of choice over this aspect of women's health. These interventions, such as abortion, sterilisation and hysterectomy are so common in this study that they have become milestones in themselves in analysis.

**Listening to the body – I'm in tune with my inner self**

Whilst discourses of health in the narrative were clearly arranged around the medical model and a relational model of health, the women also expressed an element of personal psychological health that they maintained as a monitoring system. This overview of health permeates the narrative accounts and provides the women with a way to mentally assess the state of their health, both now and previously, based on the episodes of health they have related in the account. Additionally, many of the women researched their own health in advance of the narrative interview and brought along notes. It is in this context that the women monitor, research and become experts in their own health and consequently are in a position to shape this study design by expressing how they would prefer to tell the story that they are already internally familiar with (Sixsmith & Boneham, 2003).

In philosophical terms, this represents the critical realist generative mechanism or process, by which women internalise the dynamics in society regarding health information into their health identity (Bhaskar, 1978). In narrative terms, this aligns with McAdams (1993) model of narrative identity in the context of generativity and motivation involved in the storied construction of identity. This generativity, according to Mishler, is the gift of generations in the context of generating a continuing story, which runs not only through the life story of the self, but also threads the lives of previous and future generations together. Further, personal internal monitoring is often connected with and expressed in terms of spirituality in addition to an added ideology of wellbeing that represents the psychological embodiment of health identity. Pat spoke about the way that she constantly monitors her health status, internalises health information and evaluates this in terms of her personal health:

> 'I'm in tune with my inner self...I feel my chakras spinning like a wheel, making me feel unbalanced.' (Pat, Interview 1)

Pat's internal monitoring, in common with other women in the study, suggests Descartes' (1647, in 1969 translation) dualist model has been abandoned in favour of a self-monitoring, generative mechanism that includes an interactive model of health, and that the women in this study have an awareness of this interactive model beyond the scope of mainstream health psychology as defined in the literature review in this study.

## Strong women, fragile health – Tones of narrative

The tone of the narrative account is best explored before the account is interpreted as the tone pervades the whole account (Crossley, 2000b). The women in this study told stories of a fragile health situation, but their strength in the face of adversity shone through in the tone of the telling. All of the women were optimistic about their health; many of the women had experienced serious health problems in the course of their life, but asserted that they still felt that their health had been good and were optimistic about their future health.

Lucy, a single mother who has experienced multiple miscarriages, ectopic pregnancies and suffers from stress-related depression explained that she considers herself to be healthy:

> On a scale of one to ten, ten being healthy, I would be about seven, six or seven and I do eat quite healthily and I do a lot of exercise and I drink large amounts of water but it doesn't seem to benefit me cos people around me that take well that drink coke and eat junk food seem to be just as healthy as I am. I know I'm not inside their body but they might not be as healthy but that's how it seems. But I do lead a quite healthy life style I don't smoke and I hardly ever drink alcohol. (Lucy, Interview 1)

Lucy's strength of character in her optimistic tone about health, both now and in the future, suggests that she has reframed the tone of her narrative account to deflect her bad health experiences.

When some of the women became morose about their health, it was framed as a consequence of living in a disadvantaged community in

Northern England, and they became optimistic about the ideology of escaping England to live abroad. Julie, a single parent, talked about the stress she encounters as a result of having to work two jobs and how she fainted at work through exhaustion:

> Yeah because it's like now, I think to myself. I got a mini statement from the bank this morning and I thought shit, I'm going to have to be doing overtime again this week....But anyway I'm going to save up and take me and Graham and me Mum to Spain where it's better. (Julie, Interview 1)

Going abroad, the women often felt, gave the added advantage of access to better health services.

The ideological images of future health framed in optimism pervade all the narrative accounts. The women in this study reconstructed their health identity out of health crisis towards a stoical attitude that battled against adversity. This concurs with Frank's (2000a) theory of 'narrative wreckage' and 'narrative salvage' where experiences of bad health are reframed into optimistic ideologies in order to 'rescue' the story. These women, because of their perceived disadvantage and fragile health position, have rescued their health narrative by strategising for change. This is represented by the tone of the stories and interpreted as strength in the face of the adversity of fragile health. Another strategy employed by the women in this study to salvage their narrative was to incorporate humour into their health identity. In this respect, Murray (2000) comments that:

> Bakhtin (1981) referred to the centripetal forces which pull everyday language towards the dominant discourse such that it is difficult to resist. He suggested that one way we could resist this was through buffoonery and parody. This would suggest that one way the narrator can challenge the official story of illness is through humour and mockery. (Murray, 2000, p.345)

Many of the women told amusing narratives about stories of illness and laughed when describing a health situation that was clearly painful for them. Here, Molly described her feelings about contracting hepatitis as a child and the impact it had on her family life:

> It was horrible because I was on my own in isolation unit, which was just a room with a bed and a chair and a TV. I really missed my

> sister, I missed having someone to play with and the day that I was supposed to go home the nurse came and took my temperature and then broke the thermometer on my bed and it was one of those old mercury ones and it made me vomit everywhere (laughs loudly) so I had to stay and then I finally was allowed to go home and I'd not seen my mum for ages I wasn't quite cured but they were too scared to take me back to the hospital. (laughs). (Molly, Interview 1)

Molly's experience was clearly disturbing for her and her isolation in hospital had an impact on her relationship with her family as her mother was pregnant at the time and she felt that she missed her sister. However, she deals with this by telling this story like a comedy sketch.

Similarly, Sarah, 53, told a story about painful and heavy periods that had affected her life so badly that she eventually opted for a hysterectomy, but the tone in which she told the story was jaunty and light, rushing towards a happy solution to her ill health.

Perhaps, then, the humour and playfulness in describing serious health situations found in most of the narratives are a performance of coping and strength in a time of narrative crisis. This challenges the notion of a fixed health identity as whilst the participants were often clearly distressed at the time of the health crisis, they have incorporated humour, irony and satire into their identity performance. This applied not only to past and present health but also to future expectations of health, where much merriment was made of the ageing process. In addition to this, it highlights the fragmented nature of health identity, where several identity constructing strategies are employed to rescue and salvage narrative wreckage (Frank, 2000a). The notion of a fragmented health identity is examined in detail in the following chapters.

## The storied health identity

In the next section of this chapter the considerations perimenopausal women have undergone in lived experience and how they have used these to construct and reconstruct their health identity will be explored. The considerations in this chapter are personal considerations of health, as narrated in the autobiographical accounts. This will form the first layer of the constructed perimenopausal health identity that will be modelled in the final chapter.

The narrated accounts of health were told in story form, and were fairly clearly defined in chapters and interspersed with chaotic subnarratives as described above. These chapters cover the whole of the lifespan and into future health including the perimenopausal period. This is because the design of the study aimed to capture what health considerations were important to the women, who were all perimenopausal, in terms of constructing their health identity. Analysis is based in the storied chapters of the health narrative using Murray's personal, interpersonal and ideological levels of analysis.

Identity study in mainstream health psychology traditionally uses fixed aspects of identity for the answer to the question 'Who am I?' such as 'I am a mother' and 'I am a patient'. However, in order to show how identity is constructed partially in terms of narrated health identity, which is constructed over the lifespan, such fixed labelling of identity is negated through the mutability and fluidity of interactive health identity. Murray (2000) comments that the challenge for critical health psychology is:

> ...to connect explanations across the different levels of analysis... the challenge is to connect the different levels of narrative analysis within health psychology. (Murray, 2000, p.343)

In order to avoid labelling the fragmented identity into fixed roles such as 'mother' and 'patient', the accounts were deconstructed and explained in terms of identity in action, such as 'becoming' and 'changing'. Within these actions, meaning is mutable and my analysis applies to the accounts given by the women. This helped to present the women's voices in terms of a multidirectional and fluid identity construction. Further, the use of these identity actions allows for connections across the fragmented identity, in line with Murray's comments, as the actions are interactive with each other.

The storied health identity, as told by the women in this study, was split into chapters as described above. However, the chapters were not entirely discreet from each other. Overarching themes such as resisting health, spirituality and control, and family role performance were threaded through the stories creating a smooth flow of explanation with a relational based, multidirectional timeline which constantly flitted between the past the present and the future. It is this interwoven explanation of health identity that links the stories to the perimenopause. This is because, as can be seen in the narrative accounts, health identity is constructed over the whole lived experience. So, although the stories were grounded in the present time, the narrations of health experience and its relevance to the perimenopausal health identity, that is, who the women consider themselves to be in terms of health, cover the whole lifespan. Therefore, this analysis is structured in three parts and presented it in three separate but interactive chapters. The first part, describing Narrative Touchstones of the Storied Perimenopausal Health Identity, considers the personal storied health identity and what being a healthy perimenopausal woman means, including fragmented aspects of health identity that bring meaning to storied health, and how this has been built over time. To begin this exploration of storied health and its contribution to the construction of the perimenopausal health identity, narrated personal health is introduced.

## Introduction to the personal health identity

Doise (1986) describes this personal level of identity analysis as:

> ...the theories describe how individuals organise their perception, their evaluation of their social milieu and their behaviour within this environment. (Doise, 1986, p.11)

When considering the health identity of the perimenopausal women in this study, the internal organisation and evaluation of health identity described by Doise above has been expressed through storytelling. Storytelling brings order to the chaos and confusion of health and illness and allows for self-regulation based on both internal and external constructions (Ricoeur, 1983). The health narrative, however, is not naturally divided into separate parts that express this personal consideration of health; the narrative is an interwoven mixture of personal considerations, stories of relational health identity and allusions to the impact of societal health by example of images and metaphors when the narrator is unsure of the words to use. In order to consider this personal health identity which poses the question of 'Who am I?' to women, and is answered by the story of 'Who I am', it is necessary to follow the chronology of the story itself and consider touchstones of health experiences and material health considerations that have contributed to the perimenopausal health identity.

## Health beginnings – Stories of growing up healthily

All the stories of women's health, unsurprisingly, began in childhood. Explanations of childhood health included descriptive stories of childhood illnesses such as measles, mumps, chicken pox in addition to minor accidents and ailments. However, many of the stories of health indicated the beginnings of an identity that would permeate the adult health identity and persist into the perimenopausal health identity. For example, Caroline explains her health beginnings and how these relate to her current ideas of who she is:

> The first thing I know about my health was that I was born two weeks late by caesarean because I wasn't breathing properly and erm er ... so I should have come out into my new world, my new existence much sooner than I did. And I was delayed and this seems to have been a pattern through the rest of my life. When it comes to the point where I have to do something new I go, 'Oh I don't think I can' and my mother pointed that out to me that 'You've always been a bit late'. (Caroline, Interview 1)

Caroline identifies with the lateness of her birth, which she considers an important health experience, and relates this to her adult life, giving examples of how she constructs this in who she is today. McAdams (1993) argues that recalled childhood experiences, either directly recalled or recounted by others, often set a base for the constructed identity, and in Caroline's case, these health beginnings have impacted on the construction of her identity today. Additionally, Mishler (1999) discusses life trajectories in respect of how identities are formed over time. When considering the course that the life story will take, and its impact on identity formation, Mishler recognises that the search for a 'singular, totalling identity' was not particularly useful. This was because, beginning in childhood, people's experiences are unique and therefore form unique life trajectories for identity. Therefore, the health ideas and concepts formed in childhood and lasting into mid-life, such as Caroline's lateness, shape the story of health in the future.

## Becoming a healthy woman – What health means to me

Following childhood stories of beginnings of health, the narrative account moved on to puberty and becoming. In this study women's health milestones or the uncontrollable, physiological, cyclic aspects of being a woman were both important and problematic. The physiological milestones of menstruation, childbirth or absence of childbirth and menopause provided the touchstones of experience that informed the narrative and moved the story on from one chapter to the next. These important events in the lives of women were not treated as discrete occurrences but linked with social milestones of puberty and sexuality, marriage or partnership, mid-life and ageing. Additionally, the natural milestones were overwhelmingly described as pathological, and in order to solve problems concerning the reproductive cycle, many of the participants had turned to intrusive medical intervention such as abortion, sterilisation, hysterectomy and HRT. However, on many occasions, these proved either unsatisfactory, causing women to search for alternative coping strategies, or successful in solving the physical pathology but leaving psychological problems in their wake. Stories about these milestones, whilst personal accounts of female physical embodiment of becoming a woman in the world, were inherently linked with direct relationships with the social world, their meanings illustrated by strong personal images. In this section, the narrative touchstones of experiencing menstruation and sexuality during puberty are explored.

### Puberty, periods and 'becoming'

All the women in the study talked about starting their periods in terms of a major change in their lives, about 'becoming a woman'. Linda talked about when she started her periods and the problems she encountered at that time after a healthy childhood:

> I think my mum told me when I was about ten. It must have been younger than that, about nine or ten and I started my period at eleven. I was never worried about it because my mum had explained everything to me, I suppose in a way I couldn't wait for it to happen because I knew it would be like, I'm a grown up now and I can do this, I get to use this, women products. So when it came about it was really funny because I can remember one of my friends coming up to me and happily going, 'Oh, you're a woman now.' But I had erm, went through a lot of complications, went through a lot of severe pain. I used to pass out, always being sent home from school. They'd last two weeks at a time and eventually went to the doctors and got put on medication for it. (Linda, Interview 1)

In common with other women in this study, Linda explains that 'becoming a woman' started in puberty. The expectations of this changing aspect of health identity, becoming a woman, is also highlighted in Molly's account where she explains that she compared herself with others in order to locate this anticipated construction of puberty. Tolman's (2000) work on constructs of femininity in adolescent girls supports the notion that the start of menstruation represents the beginning of womanhood and also raises the point that, for many women, becoming sexually active or considering sexual activity is also a factor in this becoming.

**Sexuality**

Two of the women in the study were lesbians, and talked about their sexuality during puberty, and the impact of this on the health milestones in their lives. Caroline talked about societal expectations in terms of women's milestones and what it meant for her:

> When it finally occurred to me that I was lesbian when I was 17 erm one of the first things I felt as terrible grief I mean terrible embarrassment, I felt 'Oh no!' mixed with a great hurray. At last I had worked out what was going on, why I don't have a boyfriend, because I don't want one, and er, but I was very, very confused. But one of the interesting things I did go through shortly after realising this was that a very strong grief that, 'Oh, so I'm not going to have children.' I made that assumption erm. And it wasn't very long but it was a sense that all the milestones had just been wiped out and looking at the landscape I was about to walk through I saw this road and I suddenly realised that there were no signposts. So there was no engagement, I know they're old fashioned stereotypical signposts but still, there wasn't any engagement, there wasn't any marriage, there wasn't childbirth so there wasn't therefore Christening which in the background I came from was the next thing after having a baby. Er, therefore there wouldn't be walks through the park with this mythical husband and pushchair. OK what am I going to do with my life? How, because I didn't have any other milestone, these are all things all women do. But er so what am I going to be doing then? No idea. In some ways it's very marvellous you realise it's a blank canvas. (Caroline, Interview 1)

Although Caroline realised that she would share the milestones of menstruation and menopause with other women, this provoked crisis in her identity in terms of her sexuality. This provided Caroline with an opportunity to reconstruct her identity, and her life, outside the societal expectations of social milestone that she was so acutely aware of suggesting that, as Mercer (1990) comments, a crisis in identity results in re-evaluation. This is in turn illustrated in the narrative as a crisis which results in the metaphor of 'a blank slate' available to Caroline for the re-construction of her identity around her sexuality.

## PMS – Feeling as if I'm a monster

The experience of a feeling of change just before menstruation, which is medicalised as pre-menstrual syndrome or pre-menstrual tension, was a recurring problem in the women's stories of health and their personal account of this, which illustrated the seriousness of this problem for women. Dell and Stewart (2000) studied the effects of hormone changes on depression and found that depression often increases under such circumstance. This study supports this suggestion from an experiential standpoint. Holly, aged 35 and has three children, talked about how PMS made her feel about herself:

> I tried self help with a healthy diet and exercise and erm that didn't seem to make a lot of difference so in the end I spiralled downwards in my emotions you know feeling as if I'm this monster, you know, it isn't going to be able to get right, there's no cure for it and I'm horrible to be with for half of the time at least. (Holly, Interview 1)

Holly's story of 'feeling like a monster' highlights the fragmented nature of health identity. As PMS is a monthly transition, Holly felt like a monster only at certain times, suggesting that this aspect of her identity is fluid. Holly's feelings and experiences when she has PMS are different to those when she does not suggest that health identity is fragmented and includes many facets of PMS identity in addition to other health concerns. Holly's negative feelings about herself eventually led to serious bouts of depression which impacted on every area of her life. Many of the women in the study expressed their concern that there was no cure for PMS and that it was outside their control. Similar arguments were made by Reilly (2000) where she notes that:

> Women's experiences which they may call PMS are a product of a multiplicity of internal and external influences interacting in complex ways. (Reilly, 2000, p.264)

The interpersonal aspects of PMS and their impact on the construction of health identity will be considered in Chapter 7.

## Building health – Constructing womanhood

The narrated health story then moved on from puberty to adult experiences of health. Whilst the participants felt that their identity now encompassed 'being a woman' in terms of passing puberty and experiencing sexuality and menstruation, pregnancy, childbirth and strategies towards wellbeing moved the story of women's health onwards. These productive aspects of identity provided the women with lived experiences that formed the building blocks for constructing womanhood.

**Abortion and the brink of adulthood – Pro-choice or no-choice?**

Fifteen women in the study had become pregnant and terminated the pregnancy. The experiences of some of the women were harrowing and this choice was clearly difficult and emotive for most of the women. Additionally, the women provided stories of mistreatment by health institutions around abortion, and talked about the psychological effects of abortion in terms of both immediate problems and more discrete problems arising later in life around issues of fertility. Kay had become pregnant due to an affair whilst she was married. She and her husband arranged an illegal abortion in order to keep the matter secret and 'save face' for her husband:

> Later I unfortunately had a fling with somebody and got pregnant and obviously I discussed it with my husband and we more or less concluded it was the other guy's child and I had an illegal abortion and that was horrendous. Not in as much as it did me any harm physically but I think it probably did me harm mentally, you know? And I thought that I would have a baby that would be disfigured and that sort of thing went through my mind. Anyway after several days it started to abort and ... Oh yeah, yeah and erm anyway it's all turned out alright physically in the end because I had two more pregnancies after that without any complications. So the next thing after that was round about '69 when I had my son who weighed 10lb! (laughs) Obviously my body was getting used to it by then, no problem there either, really healthy and everything like that and then I had another daughter in '70 and she was 10lb exactly! (Laughs). (Kay, Interview 1)

Kay's experience with the illegal abortion and her resulting problems are resolved partially in this sub-narrative changing the subject to the birth of subsequent children and by reframing the story in laughter. Kay's story contains elements of the patriarchal power dynamics in society. For Kay to put her health at risk in such a serious way in order to keep secret her affair and pregnancy to save her husband's pride, and agree to an illegal abortion which he arranged is perhaps an oppression of Kay's opportunities as a human being. Kay states that 'it all turned out all right in the end', but Kay also mentioned in the initial interview that it was she, who had decided to take part in the study because, 'I want to warn other women about illegal abortions and how they affect you for all your life...' and that she felt by telling her story to anyone she could, including me, she felt that she was warning people. Frank (2000a) provides a model for narrative salvage, where a disrupted or wrecked narrative is rescued by reframing in a story with a positive outcome. Kay's explanation of her subsequent birth following the abortion and her laughter at this salvages this narrative and restores Kay's successful construction of womanhood. However, whilst Kay has reframed her health identity through her narrative account of having children after the abortion, the action of giving the interview suggests intention towards feminist action in order to further resolve this issue for her. Alex (2004) suggests that women empower themselves after abortion by sharing stories with family and friends and this echoes Kay's experiences of deciding to share this story within this study.

### Childbirth, marriage and family – 'She was born and it was quite disastrous really...'

As the narratives progressed towards adulthood, the stories moved on to more positive aspects of women's health, such as childbirth. However, these positive and joyful personal experiences of giving birth and caring for children were often accompanied by negative experiences of postnatal depression and social issues such as economic struggle and single-parenthood that were interwoven into the personal perspective. May (2004) notes that the socioeconomic and family factors such as single parenthood produce stress in women's perceptions of their health identity, and this was reflected in this study. Julie explained that whilst her pregnancy and the birth of her son were trouble free, she suffered with various combinations of financial and family stress due to the break-up of her relationship in addition to post-natal depression. The combination of social factors such as becoming a single parent and struggling financially clearly took its toll on Julie's mental health and she was diagnosed with postnatal depression, which was compounded by the difficulties she was experiencing in her changing health identity. She had to adopt the identity of a single mother which she felt impacted on her status in her family and the community in general, leaving Julie feeling vulnerable, stressed and struggling financially.

Colleen also experienced a complex social and financial situation around her giving birth. Whilst she said that the births were fine and she enjoyed her children she also commented on how her marriage impacted on this:

> It is quite a gap, but I was very young and I didn't want any more anyway and I didn't feel like it (marriage) was working out either, and I was on the pill. I was one of the first people on the pill. I was on the pill as soon as Tracey was born and I stayed on it, and I didn't come off it until we decided to try for another baby – erm and she was born – but it (marriage) was quite disastrous really. Mainly because I felt trapped and unwanted. I was depressed. (Colleen, Interview 1)

Colleen minimised her problem by trivialising her depression, and her feeling of being 'trapped and unwanted' by her marriage which impacted on her identity and made her 'feel like I was nobody, nothing'. However, by seeking help and taking medication she became more aware of her health identity and began to feel better. The interaction of her bad marriage, taking on the extra responsibility of a new baby and the resulting depression provided a critical point in her health where she re-evaluated who she was in terms of health. However, when seeking help, she spoke about not telling her GP about her husband's cruelty and her feelings of being trapped and unwanted because she felt ashamed, just that she had depression.

Colleen's marriage eventually broke down and her depression lifted when she found another partner who cared for her. In the narrative accounts, the women describe their personal feelings about postnatal depression in context of their immediate family situation, often in terms of their partner's level of support and financial input. These accounts of building an adult health identity of womanhood were also explained in terms of successful attempts at reversing previous ill health into wellbeing.

### Wellbeing and health

All of the perimenopausal women talked about strategies they employed to stay healthy. The stories of wellbeing and health compared to a time before the perimenopause when health identity was framed in an unhealthy context with the perimenopausal health identity, where the women have strategised for health. As Roberts (2003) outlines, the storylines of narrative accounts are often multidirectional and returning to a previous point to qualify a positive change. In many cases, these were used to rationalise previous bad health and reframe their health story in a more positive light. These strategies were split into two sections: strategies to maintain good physical health and strategies to maintain good mental health.

### Personal coping strategies towards a healthy life

These stories of personal coping strategies for health highlighted meanings attached to wellbeing for the perimenopausal women, and what this means for health identity. The women in the study outlined the ways that they plan to stay healthy for the present and for the future. Some of these coping strategies were explained in terms of previous experiences of bad health and how this situation was turned around to good health, and how this was maintained. Alternatively, some of the stories were about health ideology and how, although the participant had clearly considered the implications of risky health behaviour in the light of this ideology, it proved a constant battle to comply with.

### Building a healthy identity for life

Most of the women employed strategies towards a healthy physical identity over time. As outlined earlier, the women 'listened to their bodies' in order to monitor their health status, and took steps to improve their general health. Carla, after giving birth and gaining several stones in weight, made a determined effort to get fit:

> When he (son) was five weeks old I joined the gym again. I joined this gym before we got married and then I found out I was pregnant so I didn't go again after that. I went back after the birth and I did hundreds of miles, you don't think it do you, walking along. Go back to work and be a different person. (Carla, Interview 1)

Carla's determination to loose weight after completing the childbirth milestone and become 'a different person' is an image of a drastic change in her identity as she relocates her working and fitness identities along with her identity of motherhood following the birth of her child. This symbolises Carla's embodiment of this internal change into the world, changes she hopes to build on and include in her life trajectory (Mishler, 1999).

### Building and maintaining good mental health – Walking into tomorrow

Mental health issues such as stress and depression were major themes in this study concurring with arguments made by Yardley (1997) and Ussher (1991) claiming that mental health is an important part of women's health. Whilst a further analysis of stress and depression in an interpersonal context is considered in the next chapter, many of the women mentioned personal ideology of mental health and personal coping strategies towards perimenopausal wellbeing. The women strategised towards mental health wellbeing mainly through exercise. For example, Michelle explains how she combats stress:

> If I'm very stressed I walk and I don't talk to anybody and I feel better. I tend not to confront people when I'm stressed anymore, not like 20 years ago! But tomorrows another day, tomorrows better, when I'm stressed I walk and walk into tomorrow! (Michelle, Interview 1)

Michelle's combination of positive thinking and exercise acts as a coping strategy to combat the stress in her life and the image of 'walking into tomorrow' serves as Michelle's psychological embodiment of better future health through this coping strategy. Michelle compares her health identity in terms of how she responded to stress 20 years ago with confrontation in the way she has built communication into her health strategising in order to change this to an identity of coping better.

## Constructing womanhood in terms of body image and eating behaviour

Many of the perimenopausal women mentioned that when they felt stressed or depressed they stopped eating. For some of the participants, this had led to more serious physical problems. Linda talked about how feeling depressed and stressed about being unattractive had affected her eating habits:

> I've got erm.. well, I've always had a bit, well not a problem with food but I'm always very aware of what I eat and I don't, well I try and eat healthily but I don't. I eat one meal a day and you can't be healthy eating one meal a day erm. But I do try, whereas before I just cut out meals, I don't do that any more, I mean I don't eat a lot, I do eat one to two meals a day but what I do eat, I try to make it healthy, you know I won't just go and eat a cracker or something like that (laughs) but I am very conscious and I also try and do a lot of fitness things as well. (Linda, Interview 1)

Linda's account of her change in eating patterns suggests that she has evaluated her health and the changes she has made has improved her quality of life, improving the personal perimenopausal health identity.

The transition in her eating behaviour changed her idea of herself as 'fat and ugly' and aligned her identity to health. Stopping eating in connection with jibes from other people about the body was a recurrent theme in the narrative accounts. The women in the study associated stopping eating and being thin with heightened attractiveness. Thompson and Stice (2001) and Wilcox and Laird (2000) comment on this phenomenon and warn about the detrimental effects of media advertising on women in terms of media images of women. Linda's account and the accounts of other women strongly echo this.

However, not all the accounts of building health in terms of eating behaviour were focused on body image. Often, stories that included building a caring identity in terms of health and family were told in a comparative context between the past and the present. Comments about good diet were related to a healthy lifestyle, and stories about family health in childhood included detailed descriptions of diet. Louise relates her diet today back to her childhood days:

> I mean they didn't eat terribly but I mean my Dad has a very healthy diet now. He really looks after himself but I don't know, when we were kids and I think back erm we used to eat cheese dips and pie and chips and stuff like that that I wouldn't dream of having now. Or I might have once a fortnight or...Yeah but this was like every night or whatever you know, but then again they were working and it was easy. Yeah, but in a way that's a good thing because that's what I don't do now, do you know what I mean, it sort of taught me not to eat bad, if you know what I mean? (Louise, Interview 1)

These kinds of examples of family health behaviour in the participant's childhood ties the past present and future health together. Depending on the model of wellbeing in the present (which in today's society is the 'five portions of fruit and veg per day') the past representations of family diet were portrayed as positive in Paula's narrative as it involved fruit and no takeaway food. In Linda's account of a high fat childhood diet (Anderson et al., 1998; John & Ziebland, 2004; Kelly & Stanner, 2003) it was portrayed as negative. This story about Linda as a child, in terms of healthy eating, and her healthy identity during the perimenopause when the account was narrated, shows that family health behaviour is considered as part of health identity and monitored to be held as a precedent or caution depending on the dietary trends of the present.

**Building identity by example**

The consumption of alcohol and both prescription and non-prescription drugs was discussed in many of the narratives. Most of the women talked about these in terms of the past and the effect they had on their health in conjunction with their interpersonal relationships. In most cases, these were cautionary stories that ended with consumption ceasing and recovery of health that concurs with Frank's (2000a) model of salvage of the narrative wreckage and the restitution narrative. Brenda talked about the death of her alcoholic father and her own alcoholism:

> I do come from an alcoholic family on my father's side. One or two apparently, now I find out on my mother's side but not my mother. My father was an alcoholic, two or three of my uncles were and my grandfather was so they say that dependency can be hereditary that's what I've been told. I cut down until I finally stopped drinking about three weeks before my father died. I've had the odd one since but in recent years I can honestly say I have never touched a drop. (Brenda, Interview 1)

Family stories such as this are common aspects of the narrative accounts, where vicariously experienced ill health has an effect on the health of the participant. For instance, Molly talks about how her stepfather introduced her to drugs at the age of 13, reporting that this affected her mental health most. Later in the narrative account, Molly talks about how her drug taking combined with her father's controlling behaviour made her want to escape the family and become 'another person':

> I think it impacted on my mental health in that it made me very paranoid at the time. My stepfather's behaviour towards my mum made me very paranoid that everything I did he knew what I was up to and that he'd be waiting round every corner for me so whatever I was doing at any given point I wasn't free. Erm it's scared me a lot which drove me to leave, to try and leave a lot of the time. But on the flip side of it, it drove me to be practically everything I was running away from. I became a lot more aggressive as a person and a lot more assertive erm started dressing in a more aggressive manner. Got some piercings, got myself a tattoo just anything to dissolve myself away from that family,

> be another person. Look as different from everyone I knew as I could and took a lot more drugs. (Molly, Interview 1)

Molly attempted to distance herself from her family to control what she perceived as deteriorating health, both mental and physical, and take control of her own health identity. Not only did she physically move from the family home, but she drastically changed her appearance with tattoos and body piercing to change her identity. Molly's flexible sense of identity is similar to an example provided by Burkitt (2004) when he states that:

> The sense of 'I' is established in the face of conditions that demand the flexible pliant self. (Burkitt, 2004, p.79)

Molly's early attempts to change her identity in response to unsatisfactory episodes in her life, is common with other women in this study, who typify the way women have built upon health 'beginnings' and health 'becoming' to construct strategies and tools of a fragmented health identity. These have also been the building blocks of the storied women's health so far and touchstones of experiences that have indicated narrative turns which led to the construction and re-construction of health identity. These are important indicators in the stories of the building blocks of identity that have brought the women to the perimenopause through various life trajectories. The section below follows the story of how the changing identity impacts upon health identity of the women in this study and how aspects of the fragmented identity so far have contributed to these changes.

## Changing health – Who am I now?

Following the episode of the narrative account storying building health identity and constructing womanhood, the changing nature of fertility became a consideration of health identity, as did ageing. This chapter of the women's health narrative covered the perimenopausal period and what represented the present time in storied health identity and is discussed here in terms of changing fertility identity.

### Changing fertility identity

A major change in women's health identity was the impact of sterilisation procedure on the fertility identity, and what it subsequently meant to be a healthy woman. Many of the women in the study had taken the decision to be sterilised for practical and financial reasons. None of the women had regretted this decision in the long term, but as part of their health story, discussed the difficulty around the choice of being able to have children. Louise, who has two children, went to hospital for her sterilisation procedure feeling upset about what the implications were. Here she talks about how she felt about the sterilisation and how the hospital staff treated her:

> Yeah, but when I went in last year for that they (hospital staff) were really good you know, because I was a little upset at first when I went in, because I knew I wanted it done, and I did get there and as you're going through them doors, I thought, 'This is it I'm never going to have children again.' But I knew that but I still thought it was upsetting. Yeah but they were really supportive. (Louise, Interview 2)

Louise's doubts about her sterilisation and the fact that she would not have any more children were not voiced to anyone in the hospital because she 'didn't want to be difficult' when she had arranged for the operation to be carried out. In this story, Louise's feelings were hidden from the doctor in an attempt to defend the choice she had made about being sterilised. Louise suspected that there was a shared understanding between her and the nurses that this is an upsetting time, one that is filled with feelings of sorrow at loss of fertility balanced with the choice of exercising practical control over fertility. This highlights the mixed emotions for women who choose not to have any more children and the impact on their changing identity. Yet, in considering infertility, Morse (2000) comments that the choice to become voluntarily infertile is made 'in the full knowledge and acceptance of that situation' (p.293). The women's feelings about losing their fertility through sterilisation in this study were not fully accepted at the time of the procedure and perhaps this was due to their social circumstance of living in a deprived community where to have another child would be unmanageable both financially and socially. Additionally, this highlights the intrusive nature of medically irreversible milestones; the loss of fertility through the sterilisation procedure impacts women's interpersonal narratives of perimenopause, as seen in Chapter 7.

Another medical procedure that ended fertility and affected the perimenopausal health identity in terms of womanhood was hysterectomy. The reasons for this were usually problems with menstruation, but again this often proved a difficult decision for many women. Sarah was still feeling confused about her fertility issues when she went through the final step towards the infertility of hysterectomy:

> Oh yes that's right, about that time (time of hysterectomy) I thought I was pregnant. I was 44, I had been sterilised, I was on the menopause and taking HRT but I thought I was definitely pregnant. I mean, you know what's going on with your own body, and I felt like I was pregnant. I started bleeding and I still think to this day it was a very early miscarriage. It was just an instinct, I felt completely like I was pregnant. So I went to see him and he suggested a hysterectomy. (Sarah, Interview 1)

Sarah clearly could not have been pregnant at the time of hysterectomy, but her feeling of pregnancy and her early miscarriage represented her resistance to her disappearing fertility. The transition from a fertile mother to an infertile mother was difficult for Sarah and some other women in the study. Other women talked about hysterectomy in terms of the essence of womanhood. Molly talked about her personal feelings about her hysterectomy taking away her essence of 'being female'. Here Molly mentally turns the page of her fertility story by declaring 'that chapter of my life shut' following hysterectomy. This is representative of McAdam's (1993) model of narrative psychology where the life story is naturally split into chapters and moved on chronologically. Molly's declaration moves her narrative on, not in terms of chronological age, but by a touchstone of women's narrated health; this concept is central to this study. However, she extends the medical event of her hysterectomy in a social context when she explains that it will affect not just her ability to have children, but also her chances of getting married. The social milestone of marriage was seldom mentioned in terms of the perimenopausal identity and most of the women in this study were already married or felt that their pending infertility would somehow prohibit them from getting married.

In her story, Molly's statements about femaleness resound with De Beauvoir's (1949) 'woman as womb'. This recurring theme in the narrative accounts about reproduction, fertility and the removal of the womb suggest that although women submit to the removal of the womb for medical reasons, they privately consider this as a personal loss which affects their identity as women. This was confirmed by Molly's statement that she had taken away her 'essence of womanhood' where she feels that she herself, in her choice of having a hysterectomy, had negated the previous becoming and building her womanhood in terms of health and changed her health identity into one of infertility.

## Changing bodies and hormone replacement therapy

The changing body and the embodiment of the changing health identity in the world was a major consideration in the construction of the perimenopausal identity. In this part of the health story, the participants gave a strong narrative account of their feeling and attitudes about their changing health and HRT. Most of the women in the study had tried HRT, had decided against it or held an opinion about it, implying that the issue of wellbeing during menopause is important to women (Fauconnier et al., 2000). However, many of the women stated that they would rather feel and look good during the menopause than pay attention to the risk factors involved in taking HRT. Shirley had strong views on what happens to women who are on the menopause and how HRT could help:

> But I think when you hit the menopause you know you don't become manly, but you know hair grows and your hormones change. And you have to take hormone replacement tablets. Well you don't have to but it depends what effect it has on you. Like if I reach the age of the menopause and start growing a moustache I'll be absolutely devastated and I'd run to the doctors and get HRT. I don't want my kids looking at their mum and me going seeing them graduate with a moustache do I? Like you know grey hair or big man boobs. That's my opinion, I regard my femininity as a big issue in my life and a lot of people look at me. And as far as the loss of fertility goes, that's horrific. (Shirley, Interview 2)

Shirley's concerns about HRT reveal her fear of her changing health during the perimenopausal period in terms of looking like a man. She comments that she 'regards her femininity as a big issue in my life' which suggests that her decision to take HRT is linked to her identity of womanhood and that the imminent changes during the perimenopause cause resistance in her health narrative. Kath has taken HRT and remains confused about if she has passed the menopause or not as she is reliant on the medication:

> I'm assuming I have because I've changed over onto the one which cuts your periods out. So what would actually happen if I stopped taking it I don't really know because I've been taking it for about 15 years now? (Kath, Interview 1)

Kath's perimenopausal health identity has been artificially halted by taking HRT and she felt that she 'feels fine and looks great'. However, she is uncertain about the implications of stopping HRT, perhaps fearing that the change she has tried to avert by taking it will eventually happen. Additionally, the thread of depression that Kath says has run through her life and had in fact permeated her narrative account, which has resolved itself in the perimenopausal period, and this changing health identity is one that Kath feels is of benefit. This narrative thread, that is often echoed in the narrative literature – for example by Mishler's (1999) life trajectory model and Frank's (2000a) model of illness narratives, is an important part of the autobiographical health story as it provides an identity foothold on the rocky road of the fragmented health identity. Kath is aware of the risks of HRT but is 'prepared to take a chance' to retain her identity of womanhood, feeling that she is building health by doing this. Those women who had experienced hysterectomy attached different meaning to the menopause. Clearly, after the removal of the womb menstruation had stopped. However, these women considered themselves to be going through the menopause after the periods had stopped and some had continued to take HRT for many years after hysterectomy. Deborah had a hysterectomy due to heavy periods aged 43. She explained that:

> After I had it done I was feeling a bit low, and the doctor put me on HRT. I suppose it was the menopause come early. I'm still on it now, I'm scared of coming off it in case I still have to go through the change. (Deborah, Interview 1)

It seems that the women in the study who had undergone hysterectomy still chose to experience a menopause of some kind, and take HRT even though the last medical menopausal stage together with cessation of menstruation had occurred. This suggests that representations of the menopause are so deeply entrenched in the milestones of women's health that the women in this study feel almost obliged to reach this milestone and feel that they are perimenopausal, even when this identity possibility is negated by surgery.

The overlap in the identity of building health and the identity of changing health in the narrative accounts of women's health is small but important, as it highlights the reluctance and resistance to changing health in the perimenopausal period.

Most of the women in the study, then, seemed happy to take HRT and were aware of the health risks associated with this. This attitude delaying the ageing process has been much publicised in the media and women during and after the menopause are prepared to risk their health in order to conform with a more youthful appearance. Much of this attitude is associated with expectations of the menopause and how the body changes during menopause, as highlighted in the next section.

### Changing health and the perimenopausal experience

Many of the women in the age group for this study (35–55) had experienced gradual changes in their bodies in the years leading up to loss of menses and were aware to different degrees of what to expect. All the women felt that they were perimenopausal at the time of the study. The sources of knowledge about the menopause and perimenopausal time around the menopause varied and women explained that they drew on vicarious experiences of family and friends for their understanding of what menopause is about, supporting work done by Bowles (1990), Gannon and Eskstrom (1993) and Kaufert and Lock (1997).

Women's feelings about the menopause and gradual loss of fertility leading up to its loss varied greatly. Most women expressed relief that they would no longer have periods or PMS. However several of the perimenopausal women talked about how the social aspects of their life, particularly related to their family circumstances, had contributed to negative feelings about the menopause. Michelle, aged 48, who felt that she was perimenopausal, summed up the views of many women in the study:

> Menopause? A fucking pain in the arse actually! Not looking forward to it. I don't like changes, I like things the way they are. My mum has gone through it and she went from being young and vibrant and sexual, downhill fast. My sister hasn't gone through it yet but I am now. (Michelle, Interview 1)

Murtagh and Hepworth (2003) discuss the multiple meanings of menopause for women:

> Medical and feminist descriptions of menopause posit alternative but equally-fixed truths about menopause and their relationship with the range of responses available to women at menopause. (Murtagh & Hepworth, 2003, p.185)

All the women in the study understood the medical meaning of the menopause and many of the women listed medical symptoms associated with the menopause. In addition to this, many of the women talked about psychological issues associated with the menopause such as mood swings and depression and the effects these had on their lives.

However, according to the accounts of the women in this study, other social issues of mid-life impacted on the menopause making this a difficult time for some women. Brenda told a story of her menopausal experience that involved a complex interaction of events in her life whilst experiencing perimenopause:

> My mother and she had got it over with and finished for 40 and I thought that maybe I was going to be the same but, however, my periods went right for a few years and then my marriage went wrong and I came out of the family home and started with a vengeance on the menopause because I think that stress plays a big part inthe menopause if my situation had been normal married happily situationwith teenage children which isn't easy, then I would probably breeze through it. (Brenda, Interview 1)

Brenda's story indicates that this changing health identity during the perimenopausal transition is often coupled with other competing social identities, such as becoming a wife and mother of teenage children. Brenda feels that this complicates her perimenopausal experience and draws on her inner strength to get through this difficult time for her. This tone of stoicism, as earlier coupled with difficult and fragile health experiences, are the mainstay of the narrative accounts, and Brenda's attitude of 'get through no matter what' is a thread woven through the women's accounts of health. Gail, whose husband died of cancer whilst she was perimenopausal explained that, because of the preoccupation of caring for her husband, she did not realise she was menopausal and asserted that 'I was dead thick.' (Gail, Interview 1) Gail's confusion on account of other important life events coinciding with the perimenopausal period is interesting because she transferred her experience onto the more serious and pressing issue of her husband's suffering. Gail recognised this and it's impact on her identity by commenting that she was 'dead thick' which suggests that she considers women's health and knowledge of perimenopausal issues to be related to women's intelligence and knowledge. Her omitting her own experiences into this narrative episode made her feel as if she was not intelligent and therefore lacking in knowledge about women's health, despite the understandable stress of her situation where she chose a caring identity. Both Gail and Brenda's account of the perimenopause highlight the importance and impact of ongoing family situations on the experience of the menopause. These serious narratives of mid-life that are identity crises in themselves (McAdams, 1993), are competing with those of the menopause narrative, and are consequently interconnected to health identity in a pathological way. Most of the women in the narrative accounts stated that they had received menopause information from their mothers or other family members, and as a result of this expectation of pathological perimenopause are carried through generations. This is discussed further in Chapter 7.

## Generating health – Who will I be?

The final section in the story of women's perimenopausal health experience is that of considerations of future health. Narratives of future health were concerned with musings about what women's health in old age would be like, mainly based on vicarious experiences of health in others. This is echoed in McAdam's (1993) work on the generative script, which is a narrative using the constructed identity of previous family generations to generate our own present and future narratives. Brenda considers her future health in the light of a complex family organisation and bases her generation of her own health identity on generations in her family:

> Erm like how things would be in a perfect world? Erm....Well I wish they would invent a cure for cancer. I always give to cancer charities and get my clothes from the cancer shop. Sort of to support my dad because he didn't want flowers at his funeral he wanted any money to go to cancer. Oh yes, and Alzheimer's, that's another one. My brother has it and I go to see him twice a week and oh he's wasted away, passed from pillar to post, no one can tell what he wants. (Brenda, Interview 2)

Brenda wonders if she will 'be like that' or 'will I get it' and overlays her own identity with idea of health pertaining from her father, mother and brother. When discussing her future narrative 'in a perfect world', Brenda's ideological health is based on hopes for the development of cures for cancer and Alzheimer's due to experience of these diseases through the generations of her family. McAdam's discusses this extension of health ideology through generations and Brenda's story is an example of McAdam's theorising on this. Generation of the changing, ageing identity was narrated by Sarah who talked about her ageing identity in terms of an extension of her current perimenopausal identity that included arthritis. She mentioned that despite this she intends to 'live dangerously' by continuing to smoke. Sarah's account is typical of the women in this study who frame their changing health in generating an identity based on their previous identity constructions. This has both advantages and disadvantages for women's health; on one hand, previous constructions of health identity have included fragmented aspects of identity such as building health and becoming healthy. These positive cumulative aspects of health identity bode well for a healthy ageing identity for the women. However, risk-taking constructions of perceived future health, such as smoking and 'living dangerously' suggest that other, more negative aspects of the fragmented health identity are at work.

## Conclusion

In this chapter, the personal layer of the fluid and flexible perimenopausal health identity and examined the chronological process of beginning, becoming, building, changing and generating has been covered. These fragmented aspects of the fluid and malleable health identity link narrative to identity as they both construct the narrative emplotment of the stories of perimenopausal health and describe the process by which the perimenopausal health identity is constructed. The question 'Who am I?' is asked in terms of perimenopausal health and this question is answered by providing an account of the process of personal health experiences of perimenopausal women. However, it is inevitable that this personal perimenopausal health identity will be embodied in the world in terms of health relationships in the busy lives of perimenopausal women today. In the next chapter the interpersonal aspects of lived health experience that weave together the relational health narratives are examined.

# 7
# Reaching Out – Interpersonal Narratives of the Perimenopausal Health Identity

In this chapter, an analysis of the participants' narrative accounts of health in terms of interpersonal and embodied health is presented. In the previous chapter, the women's health stories in terms of their personal and individual considerations were explored. These personal considerations looked at the touchstones of health that women used as markers to monitor their personal, individual health usually privately (but in this case they were kind enough to share these thoughts) and aside from interaction with others. This forms the first part of the layered interactive model of health identity construction that is theorised here.

In the next sections, the analysis is extended into how these touchstones of health impact on everyday relationships in lived experience. This will form a second layer of the construction of the perimenopausal health identity. Like the first personal layer, this second interpersonal layer is fragmented as it is often multidirectional and covers different aspects of identity. Again, the accounts were deconstructed and explained in terms of identity in action, this time in relational actions such as relating and performing.

## Narratives of interpersonal health experiences – He said, she said

The personal perspective of health discussed in Chapter 6 represents the reflective and reflexive health identity of the women in the study. In addition to this, as can be seen from the personal perspectives of the health identity of the women in the study, experiences of an interpersonal nature are inherent in the health experience. Earlier in this book Mead's (1934) model of identity construction was discussed where, in order to live in the social world, one has to necessarily interact with other people and this impacts on identity in a relational manner.

Murray (2000) extends the personal level of analysis in the narrative account into the interpersonal by suggesting that the narrative account is an authoring tool by which the personal health identity is shared on the assumption that it will be listened to or read. This also applies to the narrative account itself in which the teller of the tale explains how they have told the story before to others. In this study, the women qualified the narrative they gave to me by explaining how they had performed their health identity with, and to, others in examples of reciprocal health talk. This suggests that interpersonal health experiences are the situated embodiment of health identity where health information is shared in discourses of representations of health. This in turn supports representations of narrative accounts as identity construction outlined by McAdams (1993). Whilst the narratives of personal perimenopausal health formed the storyline and plot of the narrative account, and moved the plot on in an ordered temporal manner, the interpersonal narratives are multidirectional. Roughly corresponding with the personal aspects of identity in Chapter 6, and remembering and predicting health identities necessarily occurring at the beginning and end of the account, the relating, coping and performing narrative constructions of health identity overlap and pass back and forth between the personal layers of women's health identity, weaving the stories together in a relational narrative of health. In this the second part of the analysis, ways in which the participants talk of their own health experiences in relation to those of other people in terms of identity actions of remembering, relating, coping, performing and predicting aspects of the fragmented health identities are considered.

## Remembering health

At the start of the first interview, each participant responded to the first question on the interview schedule, concerning the construction of health experiences into chapters, by talking about their childhood health. Some of the participants told me that they could not remember their childhood health status and had relied on family members to give them information from which they constructed their childhood health. Roberts (2003) suggests that:

> Characteristics of the parents are passed on as part of a generational sequence, and by social transmission the cultural attitudes and values

> of the carers are carried (but not merely accepted) through socialisation, and by wider orality (Stories, myths). (Roberts, 2003, p.130)

Other participants said that they had asked their mother about their childhood illness, as only they would know what happened in their childhood. Holly recounted her childhood illness as follows:

> No its just erm trying to remember things when I was a kid, its better to ask my mum that, you know what I mean? It's like I don't know. I've heard all sorts of kids things, you know. Erm I think I had the mumps, I don't know how old I was my mum says I have and I remember having chicken pox. Can't remember how old I was either for that. (Holly, Interview 1)

Holly recounts a story of her health beginning in terms of what her mother has told her, and this negotiated account of health underlines the importance of relationships with others when constructing the health from childhood to, in this study, the perimenopause. The remembering of health from an early age is often collaborative and shaped by partial recollections filled in by family members or caregivers. The style in which Holly relates the remembering of her health beginnings is common to all the narrative accounts. All the participants reported their childhood illnesses at the beginning of the interview by listing them in medical terms, sometimes with technical language. Their reliance on the medical narrative suggests that the participants were not remembering their own memories, but what had been explained by others.

## Relating health – Family matters

As the health story progressed, narratives of relationships with others emerged. These stories were general health narratives and revolved around family situations where one or more members of a family were ill and another family member, often the participant, performed the role of the carer. Gail, who nursed her husband, talks about the effect of his illness on her own health identity:

> Then my husband started to be ill. He was ill for 10 years and he died at 50. He had bronchial asthma and they put him on steroids. They made him deteriorate and he became addicted. He was in hospital 23 times in comas. The hospital were fine but I thought he was on LSD cos he had hallucinations. They took him off all the drugs

> in the end. I piled on weight with depression and comfort eating, 17 stone, I'm only 5 foot. I struggled with my weight and the change of life. I was 48 when he died. (Gail, Interview 1)

Although Gail has heart failure herself most of her narrative account is about the health of her husband and her son and how she has cared for them by subsuming herself. The relational identity in terms of family health is clearly important to Gail, and this becomes more apparent later in the narrative when she talks about the coping strategies for health employed by her mother and her sister:

> It's been trying. But it's down to how I was brought up. My mum was very good at coping. My mum had heart trouble and she lived till she was 77. And you never heard my mum complain she just plodded on. My sister died when she was 46, absolutely crippled with arthritis and you never heard her complain. Even though she was in pain from waking up to going to sleep. My sister was a big help. People ask me how I am and I say, 'I'm fine.' My neighbours says, 'You lie, don't you?' (laughs). They don't want to know, they don't want you to mither them. (Gail, Interview 1)

Gail's stoical narrative tone is clearly a result of not wanting to appear to be unable to cope in front of other people, behaviour internalised from her mother and her sister and used to cope with her husband and her own illness. This also implies that to be in Gail's family, suffering must be borne without complaint; the family identity overrides the individual suffering. Again, this is an example of Robert's (2003) and McAdam's (1993) considerations of aspects of identity passed down through family generations. Whilst she is seriously ill and says that her life has been trying, the health identity she embodies in the world is that of 'coping well'. This internalisation of coping strategies extends from general health narratives to women's health narratives when women have to strategise for what they perceive as pathological health in all aspects of the fragmented identity. This is incorporated with the lived experience and, inevitably, relationships with other people.

### PMS and interpersonal relationships – Desperate enough to go to the doctors

An aspect of women's health that the participants experienced on an interpersonal level was a change in the days before menstruation that has been medicalised as pre-menstrual syndrome or pre-menstrual tension. Whilst PMS was also described as a personal construct of becoming a woman, the embodiment of this identity in the world and how they related to others in this context had deeper implications for how women considered themselves. As Vanselow (2000) points out, little evidence has accumulated in regard to PMS and its construction as a hormone sensitive disorder, although she comments that the media regularly report PMS as a negative experience. She also notes that future study should include 'the existence of a hormone sensitive mood disorder' (p.268). Yet many of the women in the study told graphic and harrowing stories about this and the negative effect on their interpersonal relationships and it was clearly a real problem with both material symptoms and psychological impact. Holly talked about the effect of her PMT (which is another medicalised term for PMS) and eventual depression as a result of this on her family:

> And with my circumstance being difficult at the time I think that spiralled me down into depression where I became erm depressed and dysfunctional not all the time but just a few weeks of the month so it just....But I think the root cause of it was PMT. I was trying to fight depression.

Holly explains that in trying to fight her depression, which she feels was caused by PMT, she became suspicious of her personal relationships. Holly's fighting narrative turned into a narrative of desperation and she sought medical help, but felt that her perception of herself and her relationship with her husband was affected by this. Therefore her relational identity was compromised by PMT and depression, which she felt was mostly outside her control. Relating her health identity to her partner at this time was difficult, so Holly took the step of relating her health identity in terms of PMT and depression to a health professional which improved her perception of 'why I am like it'. Additionally, some women in the study who claimed they did not suffer from PMT commented on it and recognised it as an ongoing problem for other women. Laura spoke about her not experiencing PMT but that she knew other people did:

> Oh right, I've never erm had PMT or not that I know of, erm, no, I don't think I do no. I think I'd probably know about it if I did.... I'm quite lucky really, I suppose I shouldn't really whinge I mean some women go through all kinds of hell, but I keep thinking I might have to develop PMT sometimes. I don't know what to do you see,

> maybe you could give me some pointers? Hints and tips on a premeditated tantrum, yeah. That's what Sid calls it, premeditated tantrum. (Laura, Interview 1)

Laura touches here on the negative imagery of PMS and PMT by adapting the acronym PMT to 'premeditated tantrum'. What Laura sees as quite a serious health problem is turned around to a mocking attitude to the exclusively female affliction, which is often observed in the popular media and by men who do not directly experience PMT. Because she does not suffer from PMT, Laura has adapted her husband's view of PMT as 'premeditated', and even though this was treated with humour, this negative attitude towards ill health experienced exclusively by women such as PMS, PMT and the menopause is common (Rostosky & Travis, 1996) whereas genderless general health is treated more seriously. This suggests a patriarchal view of women's health where some men see women's reproductive health as trivial and an excuse for manipulation of the expectations of the role of women.

### Perimenopause and interpersonal relationships – He'll just squeeze me so tight and I'll probably cry

The perimenopause and its social construction were discussed at length in the narratives. The women who considered themselves perimenopausal gave detailed accounts of how menopausal psychological symptoms such as mood swings and mental tiredness, and physical symptoms such as irregular periods and general tiredness affected their ability to cope both in family life and at work. This details the transition from building a health identity to a changing health identity as detailed in the previous chapter. Cynthia, who says she is currently on the menopause and experiencing mood swings, talks about how her mood swings affect her relationship with her husband:

> I said to Stu, 'Just read those passages' and he said, 'Oh have I got to put up with all this? ' So I told him he had two choices! (Laughs) All he does if I start shouting and banging, I bang, he'll come in the kitchen and get hold of me and hug me so tight and he'll just squeeze me so tight that I'll probably cry and then I calm down. So I'm just glad that I've got him. Because I talk to some women at work and there's two others on the change besides me, one's only forty six, and she's on the change and she doesn't discuss it with her husband at all, you know she's left him twice, and I say talk to him, sit him down and talk to him. He looks at me and he'll say, 'Go on,

> get it out!' there's a lot you couldn't do it with, my friends husband Geoff he loves her to bits but he doesn't want to know. Its not because he doesn't love her, it's because he can't understand what she's saying to him. (Cynthia, Interview 1)

Cynthia clearly describes the perimenopausal transition as 'the change', supporting notions of the fragmented health identity constructed in the light of changing health in this book. Cynthia compares her experience of the menopause, and how it affects her close interpersonal relationship with her husband, with that of her friends and colleagues. She asserts that although she cannot help her behaviour, her good communication with her husband, (which includes providing him with books and pamphlets about the menopause) has improved his understanding of her unpredictable behaviour. This is an example of cross gender understanding through which the narration of the relational health identity emerges in terms of understanding. Cynthia stresses the importance of understanding in her narrative accounts and how this facilitates the smooth transition of her changing health identity. Additionally, Sarah, who has since had a hysterectomy to deal with menopausal symptoms revealed how her physical symptoms made even the most normal everyday tasks with her children difficult:

> I mean I would never try to talk anyone else into it, but I couldn't cope with the kids like that. One Saturday I took them dancing and I had to come home and get changed, the blood just soaked into the car seat and all my clothes. And I never knew when it would happen. (Sarah, Interview 1)

Sarah found it so difficult to cope that she had a hysterectomy on the advice of her doctor, and suffered psychological problems following this regarding her loss of fertility. It is clear from these accounts that the changing identity during the perimenopause is a difficult time for women, and many of the women felt that talking to someone about this time in their lives was beneficial. Cynthia went on to say that:

> Talking to you and explaining every part about it because nobody does ever listen. (Cynthia, Interview 1)

The main theme of those women who considered themselves to be perimenopausal was lack of information or information that did not correspond to how they were feeling. Many of the women looked to their mothers as their major source of information but as Michelle points out:

> Yeah, she went through it OK, had hot sweats and all that, was a bit moody, never really said how she felt but sometimes you could just see it in her. She looked like she wanted to kill someone and I suppose if she didn't know what was happening to her and what these feelings were, how could she tell us? (Michelle, initial interview notes)

Michelle's experience of lack of information from her mother in their health relationship impacted on her changing health identity in terms of building health. Without this point of reference from her mother about approaching menopause and what it involves, her health identity during her own changing transition was compromised due to lack of an appropriate relationship within which to build expectations of the changing health identity during the perimenopause. This again highlights the importance of the interpersonal relational health identity for women.

## Coping with health – Understanding and support

The fragmented health identity of perimenopausal women included aspects of understanding and support from others in terms of health. In times of narrative crisis the women presented a clear narrative of coping, which included reciprocal caring of health relationships. All of the narratives contained at least one story about the ill health of another person and how this impacted on the health of the participant. Most of the other people discussed were family members or close friends. Each story was framed in terms of 'lessons learned' and included explanations of strong emotions and feelings that were largely absent from the stories of personal health in Chapter 6. These interpersonal experiences of health contribute to the perimenopausal health identity in that they presented the participants with an opportunity to experience the performance of health behaviour, positively or negatively, of another social actor and internalise this into their own health identity (Goffman, 1959). The performance of health behaviour by others made an impact upon the participants as they explained these in terms of not only the health of the person involved, but in terms of its effect on their own health and how the health problem was resolved (Adams, 2000). In this section, the ways in which women cope with stress and depression in the light of their personal relationships and their relationships with health-care providers is examined. The narratives of the social nature of health, support and understanding in terms of coping were clear and sometimes painful and upsetting for the participant to recall.

### Stress, depression and interpersonal relationships

Whilst stress and depression were described in terms of personal health events in the previous chapter, the way that these were embodied in the world provided different narratives of reciprocal coping strategies. These in turn embodied a coping identity that permeated the narrative accounts. Stress and depression played major roles in the health lives of women in the study, a view often echoed in women's health literature (see Stoppard, 2000 and Lawthom, 2000). Most of the women who claimed to be stressed said that this was an ongoing problem, often due to problems with their finances or personal relationships. The women who had suffered from depression told stories about major life events such as death of a loved one or divorce that had left them depressed. However, the participant often did not associate the relief of stress and depression with changes in their ongoing personal relationships, but turned to other coping strategies as 'cures'.

### Coping with stress

Feelings of stress were reported by most of the women in the study at some point in their lives. Many of the perimenopausal women felt stressed about family situations whilst some felt stressed about money. Often the women spoke of stress in terms of a personal feeling embodied in the social world through their ability to deal with the situation that caused them stress and physical symptoms of stress combined. Carla's account of stress caused by her baby having chronic eczema and not sleeping at night is an example of the impact of stress on interpersonal relationships.

> It's the sleep deprivation that did it I think. I love me kip! Every night we'd get him to sleep and he's go to bed about 8 o'clock and we were pottering about making buttys for the next day and we'd go to bed about half ten, eleven. We never row, we don't argue at all, he's dead placid but we were just screaming at each other all the time. Like it was his fault and he'd shout at me like it was my fault. I feel knackered now just talking about it. I woke up that morning when he had slept through, I woke up with my alarm clock and I woke up and I said, 'Shit Dan, Sam hasn't woke up!' We thought

> maybe he'd got up in the night and we hadn't heard him. We both legged it into his bedroom and he was asleep. And we had to wake him up. (Carla, Interview 1)

The combination of sleep deprivation, stress and perimenopausal symptoms eventually caused Carla to lose her job, throwing her work-life balance into chaos and causing further stress provoking financial problems. Carla went to the doctor for help for her son's eczema and her stress and says that her GP 'just didn't listen'.

Carla's lack of confidence in her GP, which is a common thread throughout the narrative accounts, may be due to lack of communication and lack of understanding of the holistic nature of stress problems, particularly the stress of those who care for the chronically ill. This stressful time for Carla, which occurs whilst she is approaching the menopause and with a small, ill child to care for highlights a combination of problems in lived experience that contribute to a negative perimenopausal experience.

## Coping with depression

Coping with depression was also a recurrent theme in the narrative and dominated some of the perimenopausal women's lives. Whilst talking about depression in terms of personal feelings, the women always related their own depressed feelings to how this affected their lived experience, particularly the impact of their depression on family members. Sometimes this effect dynamic was a reciprocal situation, where the participant became more depressed because of the effect of her depression of other people who she perceived as causing her depression. At other times, the participant would examine the support network within the family in terms of her depressed behaviour. Holly describes this in detail:

> Well the first problem was getting it diagnosed because you just think that well you know you think that its your relationship because you start falling out a lot and having big bust ups and I thought it was the other person, you are the person saying, 'Hang on what's going on here with this person?' And eventually it came to a head where I was desperate enough to go to the doctor and say that I was so desperate and he recognised the symptoms and said he would start treating me for depression, you know, I saw a psychiatric community nurse I think it was and talked things through and that helped. Erm went on a course of anti depressants and erm they helped a little bit. Just getting more understanding about my condition and erm

> why I was like it and stuff was a big part of getting over it. (Holly, Interview 1)

Holly's narrative account detailed her struggle with depression and the way she related with her family and carers during this time. Without the understanding of others in her personal relationships, which was compromised by her medical condition, Holly turned to a healthcare relationship for help. These relational coping strategies are important to the women in the study who suffered stress and depression and have been explored further in the next section.

### Coping strategies for stress and depression

The women who were stressed or depressed had usually visited their GP to get help for this problem. However, they often refused medication and employed other coping strategies to combat these health problems as discussed below in terms of relaxation.

### Coping and medication solutions – Just relax, you don't need those

The experience of stress and depression by the women is a major problem in the lived experience for the construction of health identity. This crisis in the narrative account was described in detail and in context of the social situation of the women. The women attempted to address this problem by visiting their general practitioner with varying results. In many cases, the women who visited their GP did not get time to explain the complex social conditions that they felt contributed to their stress and depression, or felt that they did not trust their GP with this information. The resulting stories describe the women's feelings regarding the prescribing of anti-depressants and their attitudes to this. Cynthia describes a visit to her doctor's following a panic attack at work and reported that the blood pressure tablets she was prescribed turned out to be anti-depressants, a fact not communicated to her by her GP.

Cynthia spoke about how she did not tell her GP about failing to take the tablets following this incident because she no longer trusted her. Brenda was prescribed medication by her GP. She said that:

> So all in all things started to even out a bit more still some depressions still to this day on what I call my brain tablets but are actually called ventoflaxin erm quite a strong dosage and they do keep me. I know I couldn't take them one day because of sickness and erm I could tell I hadn't taken one because I was really down. Anyway it

> just shows you that modern medicines have improved and that things can be changed by them. Before counselling I was put on Serroxat I don't really know much about these kind of tablets it's just that I always read the leaflet that come in the boxes. I wasn't thrilled at being on them. They are for depression serroxat and erm. Oh I was on these for years and then about four years ago this is when I came up to the age of 51 my brother was diagnosed with Alzheimer's disease....Erm, I started to feel myself going very down again and I'm still on the serroxat so I went back and told my doctor. He sent me to another psychiatrist. (Brenda, Interview 1)

Brenda's experience of depression and medication involved a lengthy trial and error of different medications, counselling and psychiatric assessment. The complex family situation that Brenda faced at this time made her life difficult, in conjunction with her transitional perimenopause, her depressive condition negated her ability to adopt a coping identity, and consequently she began to take anti depressants. However, Brenda commented that she had not explained the complex family situation surrounding her condition to anyone she had consulted as she felt that it was not relevant to her condition in medical terms. This has led to an over-reliance by Brenda on medication for depression, and Brenda's coping strategies for depression are focused on repeat prescription, provided by her GP without consultation on her social problems.

### Coping and alternative remedies

An alternative strategy employed by the participants to alleviate stress and depression was the use of alternative remedies. The women in the study told stories of how they had researched this area through social networks, the internet and books. This proved a successful strategy, particularly when visiting an alternative therapist, when the women thought that they were listened to and were given more time to explain. Tina told a story about her visit to the homeopath to solve her depression problems:

> I went to a homeopath twelve months ago actually cos I was so down and depressed and my son's girlfriend is training to be a homeopath, we're all into homeopaths, all my family's into homeopaths, and I went to see her, Catherine she was called, for two hours and I told her everything, all my life story, I went through everything, and she was superb, absolutely super. When I came out of there I felt like I had a big cloud lifted off my shoulders. Two weeks after

> she sent me a remedy, two little tiny tablets, and I was great, I was absolutely, no depression, I was happy, everything. (Tina, Interview 1)

Molly tried alternative remedies for depression and stress related to PMS with less success.

Molly found no real relief in alternative remedies and through trial and error found that, her own coping strategy of relaxation techniques helped her most in her health crisis. This trial and error testing of different ways of coping is representative of Frank's explanation of life trajectories in that Molly was trying to change her negative experience of health to a positive experience, and tried many potential new life trajectories before finding a coping strategy that she felt she owned. This further suggests a fragmented health identity in terms of Gergen's (1991) postmodern saturation of society with a multitude of fragmented possibilities to consider. She commented, however, that had she not experimented with alternative medicines and therapies, she would not have found out about relaxation therapy, and would have 'ended up on anti-depressants'.

### Coping using intoxicants – You only live once!

Alcohol and drugs were an important aspect of a sense of wellbeing. The women in the study stated recurrently that they used drink and drugs socially, including nicotine, as stress relief, and although they realised that this was risky behaviour they felt that this was a valid coping strategy. Julie clearly states that she uses alcohol to 'chill out' when she feels stressed, but tells a story full of imagery about her recognition of what harm this could do to her:

> I chill out, have what I want to eat, have a bath then probably have a drink, you knew that would come in somewhere didn't you! (Laughs) You know because you've got to do, don't you, you have to chill out. I was sat there and my mate Margaret looked at me and she said, 'Are you all right?' and I went 'No!'. And I was sat there on this stool in the Grey Horse and I went, 'I don't feel real!' (Laughs) And I said, 'I need to go to the toilet!' And she said, 'Well go!' She came into the toilets Margaret and she said, 'Make yourself sick!' and I said, 'I've got my fingers down my throat.' (Laughs) I couldn't make myself sick for the life of me. I thought 'I can't do this!' And I came out and all my make up had run. Cos of the tears and everything and she said, 'Right, you're going on water!' So anyway she got me a glass of water from the bar, I drunk that and right as rain! I said, 'I'll have another brandy and coke now!' and she said, 'You bleeding won't! But you've got to go out

> every now and again and let your hair down. You only live once! That's my de-stresser anyway. (Julie, Interview 1)

Julie's story about drinking to alleviate stress illustrates how, to cover any serious risk analysis that occurs pertaining to this behaviour, the story is framed in a humorous tone. The comedy images and language used make what is clearly an impact on Julie's health with humour. This is an example of Murray's (2000) buffoonery tone, which in the health narrative is often used to detract from the dominant discourse of the danger of intoxicants in order to make Julie's use of alcohol as a de-stresser acceptable in the narrative. Other participants spoke about using illicit drugs to alleviate tension and stress but also stated their worries about the long-term effects of this risky behaviour on their future health. Ruby, who had experimented with drugs in her teens and early twenties, said:

> I used to smoke a bit of weed to help me relax and now and again would have some LSD or speed, just recreational uses, erm, but they helped me to enjoy myself at the time. I don't do it now because of the kids, but I think I would if I didn't have them. Yeah it's just, well that, well you don't know what it does to you? No one knows what the long term effects are of drugs do they? I do worry about it. But it was so relaxing at the time, like all my worries went away for a bit. Nothing seems to have happened to me yet, but I do worry. (Ruby, Interview 1)

These risky behaviours, which, in terms of stress have positive outcomes for the women, also carry more risky implications for health in general. In critically evaluating the health identity construction of the women in this study, it is worth noting that the possibilities for these women to take drugs and drink alcohol in social situations may be indicative of lived experience of a deprived environment, with desperate measure being taken to alleviate the increased stress level of, say, single parenthood or economic instability.

## Performing health – Getting on with it

Within the fragmented health identity lie representations of family roles, and roles involved in being a woman. Performances of these roles were important to the women in this study on an interpersonal level, and much of their health identity is invested in these roles. However, these role expectations worked in a multidirectional manner concerning health. Whilst the performance of the role identities concerned with family relating relied on good health, using health as an excuse for not performing these fragmented role identities featured in the narrative constructions of coping.

**Health as an excuse**

In particular, some participants talked about the health behaviour of their father or mother when they were children, and related it to their health behaviour today. This 'returning' is outlined by Roberts (2003) in his explanation of narrative timelines, which he suggests are not strictly chronological in one direction, but can be chaotic in nature. Many of the participants were emotive about the way they felt their parents manipulated their health status in order to avoid taking part in family activities, such as childcare or work around the house. In some cases, this influenced the participant's own health identity, making them ignore their illnesses so as not to be seen as using health as an excuse. Shirley spoke about how she recognised this avoidance through making health an excuse in her family:

> You know even when I remember my sister had a termination and lay on the bloody settee for three weeks. I had one and I was in the pub the next day. Because I didn't feel it necessary to go, 'Woe is me' and be a martyr. That's what happened, that's the decision I made health wise I was fine mentally. I might not have been but I got up and got on with life, cos that's what you've got to do. Can't sit around and be a martyr and you can't sit around and expect everyone to wait on you hand and foot and you can't use health as an excuse either to not do things. Like you know, Oh I'm ill I can't do this really important thing or you know I don't want to see you, I haven't seen you in ages but....' My grandma's like it. But I don't think I'm like that. I hope that I've rebelled against the norm. It's like the man who cried wolf. (Shirley, Interview 1)

The symbolism in this extract is important as it links with a well-known metaphorical story from folklore. Shirley defends her position of 'rebellion' by citing an example from a different narrative as an example of her opposition to the behaviour pattern in her family of using health issues to avoid tasks that they do not wish to do. This imagery points to a moral crisis in Shirley's identity where she looks outside the family to reconstruct her identity in the light of a firm moralistic story about the man who cried wolf. She 'gets on with life' and adopts a coping identity formed through the antithesis of her perceived family role, health identity, and the way it was manipulated.

In other cases, this influenced health identity in another way that aligned it with their parents' behaviour of avoiding situations through a stoical attitude to health. Caroline based her health identity construction on her father's austere attitude to health in contrast to her mother's avoidance of the family using health as an excuse:

> So you know we didn't get, well, very often I was sent to school when I was ill even though my mother didn't have a job. It was just like well, you know, we don't just lie down. I think that came from my stepfather. We don't lie down we just carry on. Very public school attitude. Erm and er yeah, so it wasn't a prompt for loads and loads of love and affection from my mother. She used to say 'Oh I'm getting ill, I'm so ill' and have to go to bed and wanted to be very much looked after. It was part of a larger, larger syndrome but we definitely had the idea that it wasn't alright if we needed lots of care and attention to be ill, but if she was the slightest bit ill she needed lots of attention, so...mmmm. (Caroline, Interview 1)

Caroline sees her construction of health based on her father's stoicism as a strength as opposed to 'weakness to get ill' and this is linked to the tone of her and other narrative accounts of strong women in fragile health situations.

Health as an excuse for seeking attention or as an excuse to avoid domestic chores in family life was a common theme throughout the narrative accounts. The participants often gave examples, like Shirley and Caroline, of their mothers or sisters or grandmothers using ill health in order to make themselves unavailable for the role expected of them in the family; this often involved taking to their bed. There was a general assumption of disbelief, that the illness was either manufactured or exaggerated in order to avoid having to state directly that they did not wish to take part on the role that was expected of them in the family, at least on a temporary basis. This suggests that the patriarchal model of the family (Coser, 1977) was so demanding for these women that they could not, for fear of shame and guilt, simply state that they did not choose to fulfil the role expected of them at that time, and would use health as an excuse to make themselves unavailable. Conversely, in exaggerating illness in order to draw attention to themselves, the women embodied illness in a way which feigned helplessness in order to receive emotional contact with the family in a way which was normally smothered by their expected role.

Both these examples suggest a struggle to escape a role identity so constricting (De Beauvoir, 1949) that manipulative behaviour was required as an avoidance technique. In observing this behaviour and recognising the manipulative nature of such, the participants clearly stated that they endeavoured to amend their health identity into a more stoical model performance in the role of 'get up and get on with life, cos that's what you've got to do.'

## Predicting health – Ending up like my parents

In contrast to the reporting of listing in medical terms, a different picture of childhood health appeared later in the narrative, again concurring with Robert's (2003) theory of chaotic storylines. When talking about their future health, the participants' related stories about health behaviour in the family during their childhood. These anecdotal stories about how their parents safeguarded the childhood health – or not – were in more detail than at the start of the narrative and occurred in the closing sub-narratives of the first interview. Kath, who listed various childhood illnesses at the beginning of the narrative, talked later in the account about having a facelift.

> I don't know if this is relevant or not, round about the same time I had a face lift. I always had it in the back of my mind. I know its going to sound horrible this but I didn't want to look like my mother. So I think that was my main motivation really. Yeah, yeah. I'm determined not to be as difficult as my mother was. Oh yeah, bloody hell yeah. Very erm really. But very manipulative really. She more or less erm was diagnosed with a personality disorder which I don't suppose she could help. She made my life a misery and my dad's life a misery. Full stop. Which was probably why I was the way I was, you know, depressed as a kid and stuff like that. You don't realize when you're a kid do you, its only when you look back how everything looked black and stuff like that. She really wasn't easy, and she died a couple of years ago. My mother and father died within a short space of time. It was really hard. I seem to be able to deal with situations for some reason, and I don't know why. But she was still hurting me up until her dying. Nothing serious, but a quick back hander if I didn't comply with. (Kath, Interview 1)

The impact of her mother's mental health problems in her childhood, which led to depression through her whole life, led Kath to go to great lengths to not be like her mother. This suggests, as others have outlined (McAdams, 1993; Mishler, 1999), a discontinuity in the narrative account that Kath felt she had to address before she could look forward. Kath's pain extended to changing her appearance with plastic surgery so she would not look like her mother who was the embodiment of what she considered ill and unhappy. As a result, Kath's narrative account exemplifies the past, present and future relationships with her health identity and allows her to predict her future health with more certainty. Her experiences in her past, with her mother's and her own crises with depression and her decision to change not just her health identity on a psychological level, but her physically embodied identity to the world, cast this new health identity construction into the future representation of how Kath feels her wellbeing, in terms of health, can be constructed. This multidirectional timeline is similar to Ricoeur's (1985) defence of history as fiction. Ricouer argues that all history is fiction because the retelling of the story is an attempt to fictionalise events of the past and either over or underplay narrative events with the motive of reframing them in positivity. Kath has recognised that although she remembers her past in a negative context her embodiment of herself in the present and the future as someone different to her mother's daughter has enhanced her wellbeing and turned the past into a positive catalyst for change. As each moment passes and Kath's new identity reinforces itself, the near past overwrites the far past and merges into a reframed fictional account which is subject to change based on her future perceived narrative and as a consequence, predictive. In another narrative account, the issue of adoption was raised. This made it difficult for the participant to have knowledge of predicted future physiological health in terms of family history. Holly, when asked about her expectation of future health said:

> Well the big thing I've got there is with being adopted I don't have any big medical history as such. And sometimes I think that can be a positive thing cos if there was any problems then you've got something to worry about but on the other hand there are things that I could be screened for. But if I'm not aware of my medical history then there's nothing there to give me any clues. Erm I mean often when you're at the doctors and that they ask you if there's any history of heart disease or whatever in your family and I don't know. So that could leave me vulnerable and erm as a child but not so much now at the back of my mind is always the fear of cancer. And I think if there was a history of a certain kind of cancer in my

> family then there's no way of me knowing about it. No way of me getting any extra screening if I should, so that is a bit of a worry. (Holly, Interview 1)

In Holly's perception of her future health, she is not able to take advantage of information about family health problems passed on through the family network, as she has no knowledge about her biological family. This highlights the importance of uncertainty in predicting her health outcome and constructing her health identity. Her lack of information about the past has led to uncertainty about her future health reconstruction in the light of health risks. However, health behaviour concerning the adoptive family and the impact of this on the participant's life was still widely discussed in the narrative account. Although Holly did not have any information about her birth mother or father, the social nature of her adoptive family's health had an impact on her future health expectations, for example, she commented that:

> Yeah, me Nan when she got Alzheimer's and I suppose one thing I can be thankful for is that I don't have her genes. You know I'm adopted so obviously she's my adoptive Nan. So erm I look at some of the things that probably triggered her Alzheimer's, aluminium in her system could be a factor. She cooked with aluminium saucepans and she was forever taking indigestion remedies containing aluminium so that one of the things I know to watch for. I keep away from stuff like that. That's something that I would definitely not like to happen. (Holly, Interview 1)

This suggests that Holly is personally generating and interpersonally predicting her future health identity. Despite her lack of information from her birth parents, Holly still relies on interpersonal relational narratives about her adoptive parents to predict her future health identity.

## Health and relational identity – Images and metaphors as signposts and interactive themes

As can be seen from the personal and interpersonal identity actions in the previous two chapters above and the narratives of the participants, personal health and interpersonal health are closely combined in the construction of health identity. The participants, whilst having a clear idea of their own storied health, exhibit a relational element in constantly modifying their health identity by considering their own experience and the health experiences of others.

This relational construction of health identity on an interpersonal level involves mainly social encounters with the health behaviour and physiological health status embodied in the world by other people. As can be seen in this chapter these encounters have an impact on future health behaviour. This also illustrates how stress, depression, and the coping strategies employed to deal with them affect not only the person experiencing the ill health, but also other people around them. The strong images and metaphors involved in the telling of the stories illuminate the social experience and are quite explicit signposts to the importance of 'the other' in the embodied health identity.

However, society consists of not only interpersonal relationships with other people, but also institutional power dynamics that are more implicit in shaping society and the individual. In order to take a critical approach to the study of identity construction of perimenopausal women it is necessary to examine the societal overarching aspects of the fluid and fragmented health identity. This is important for the construction of perimenopausal health identity as social, cultural, and political power dynamics compete for ontology and truth in the health society in today's globalised society. In the next chapter, the impact of various societal discourses in terms of institutional power and ideology and investigate where the women's health identities are located in these will be examined.

# 8

# Stories of Societal Health – The Impact of Narrated Positional, Situated and Ideological Health Representation

In this chapter, health representations in society in terms of the women's narrated accounts are examined in order to critically analyse how positional and ideological societal representations of health are situated in the perimenopausal health identity. In the previous chapters two layers of the perimenopausal health identity construction have been theorised, the personal layer where individual considerations about health are explained in terms of touchstones of health and an interpersonal layer where relationships with others are examined in terms if identity actions such as performing and relating.

In the following sections several aspects of positioning and situations in society are considered and how ideological representation of health from institutions such as healthcare organisations and the family impact on the construction of health identity. Again, this layer of the perimenopausal constructed health identity in terms of actions instead of roles is analysed here, as this represents a fragmented identity that is fluid. This is particularly important in societal terms as the saturation of society by opportunities for individuals to encounter health representations is complex (Gergen, 1991). A fluid and mutable health identity would be necessary in order to accommodate this saturation and the accompanying rapid movement in health technology. The construction of the perimenopausal health is therefore examined identity in terms of identity actions such as controlling and returning so as to emphasise the interactive nature of these with the previous layers of health explained in Chapters 6 and 7.

## Belonging and health – A time and place

In order to take a critical approach to the analysis of construction and reconstruction of perimenopausal health identity social and cultural aspects of health are considered here. This clarifies the social and cultural shared meaning of health and any financial and power inequities in the environment surrounding lived experiences of perimenopausal women. These aspects have been explored according to Murray' positional and ideological level of analysis. Murray (2000) comments that:

> It is through the sharing of stories about illness, that a community creates a mutually intelligible world. As such, investigation of narratives informs us of the cultural assumptions that permeate our society and our very identity. (Murray, 2000, p.343)

It is therefore necessary to investigate the social and cultural assumptions that perimenopausal women have undergone throughout their lifespan in this study in order to broaden the context of their health identity today. In Chapter 6 regarding the personal narratives of women's health, the fragmented health identity was discussed, and the idea that these sub-identities (Frank, 2000a) may either align or conflict with each other. In this positional and ideological level of analysis, aspects of the perimenopausal health identity in society that may cause identity conflict will be considered. So far, in this story of the autobiographical health of perimenopausal women, the personal and interpersonal layers of identity have caused little conflict in their interaction, and the women have been able to salvage the narrative when conflict has occurred. The final ideological and positional layer, however, holds concepts of power, difference and control in society that are signposts for ideological notions of good health. In this study, and partly due to the disadvantaged social positioning of the women, the conflict in identity arises when ideological representations of health mismatch with the personal and interpersonal narratives of lived experience.

The women in this study were recruited by a newspaper advertisement that appeared in the town's free newspaper and was therefore distributed to everyone in the town. Initially there was an overwhelming response to the advertisement for women to take part in the study, but this was narrowed down to 32 women by eliminating those outside the age range and the completion of a participant pack which outlined the level of time commitment needed to take part in the study. During the initial meeting, the interviews and debriefing interviews, none of the women told me that they were feminist or spoke about feminist ideals. However, the fact that women responded to an advertisement, which appealed for women's voices about health, suggests that in an implicit level feminist theory may be at work. The women took action to make their voices heard and invested time in this action, the very premise of turning a feminist epistemology to feminist ontology. It is on this basis that this study has empowered these women. This was clearly reflected in the following comments:

> The study has made me conscious of all health issues on a day to day basis. It has been a good thing as we are making changes to our daily lives now to improve health – especially where the kids are concerned. (Sandra, Study Notes)

> This study has made me realise just how relaxed and possibly carefree I have been about my health – I don't have many worries, but it's highlighted the need to care for myself better, especially regarding exercise. This will help me a lot in a few years in a positive way. (Laura, Debriefing)

This is an example of implicitly feminist action that may have led to positive changes in the health identity of the woman concerned. Because of the circumstances of living in a disadvantaged socially and economically deprived community, time and place are important considerations in these narrative accounts. Sixsmith and Boneham (2003), in their study about single mothers in a deprived community, comment that:

> ...health is very much tied into women's everyday community based lives and sense of identity. (Sixsmith & Boneham, 2003, p.245)

This view was supported in this study by Julie and Cynthia's stories in Chapter 6 which detail their lack of trust in local health facilities and both wanted to emigrate to Spain because of this. However, although place is important in identity, a sense of taken-for-granted attitude towards life in a deprived community was present in most of the accounts. The women had mostly lived in Oldham, a disadvantaged community in Northern England, all their lives and although some said that they would like to move abroad, none of the women had made plans to move away. Work by Taylor (2004) on place of residence in women's lives suggests that place identity is particularly meaning-making and that 'belonging to' one community for a long time without moving away strengthens place identity. In the research detailed in this book, the women's stoical tone (Chapter 6) and their assessment of themselves as 'strong women' is very much based in the place they have lived for so long. In the face of the adversity of social deprivation and resisting health problems, both material and socially constructed, the women have adopted strength of identity that reflects their fight for health; this is represented as conflict in the fragmented health identity. Many of the women referred to negative aspects of their everyday community living in connection with their health in the narrative accounts. As discussed earlier in this thesis, the government has devised a measurement of deprivation through the Indices of Deprivation Report (2004). This is made up of seven domains which are identified by government agencies as problematic in society. These are: income deprivation; employment deprivation; health deprivation and disability; education, skills and training deprivation, barriers to housing and services; living environment deprivation and crime. These domains are interactive in the measurement of deprivation and are political in the sense that decision-making power lies with government agencies for matters that effect women in everyday life. In the narrative accounts, most of the issues that these domains were concerned with were mentioned. For example, Molly, a single parent, talks about her barriers to housing services by explaining how she became homeless and had to sleep on her ex-partner's floor due to the local council decision to not let her have alternative accommodation when she was robbed and scared:

> Well I had two children and I went to live in a council house for three weeks and couldn't handle it...The locals picked on me and tried robbing my house. Breaking into it while I was in and I ended up going living back at my mums which was a wee bit stressful because we had not lived together for years and she was like sorting her life out...me and my mum ended up having this colossal row with me leaving with a bin bag full of stuff. In true Mary fashion (laughs) and going staying with my son's dad and his fiancé, all of us sleeping on the floor, which was a bit bizarre and shortly after that, a couple of weeks before Christmas, I moved into my own house. I rented a house. Cos they wouldn't let me have a council house coz I had made myself intentionally homeless, they called it and I didn't have a job. (Molly, Interview 2)

This domain of deprivation clearly interacts with the crime domain, as Molly suffered from crime committed which in turn caused her to be homeless, the health domain as Molly became severely stressed, and the income and employment deprivation domains. This pattern of interaction of the domains of deprivation interacting with the health domain is repeated in all the narrative accounts and highlights the importance of health identity when considering social deprivation.

## Social deprivation and personal identity

In the analysis of the narrative accounts, health-focused issues in the women's accounts affect all of the domains of deprivation. These domains of deprivation work interactively with each other and are not discreet categories. The domains of deprivation seem at first glance to fit well with Fox and Prililltensky's notions of critical issues and indeed appear to correspond with issues critical psychology addresses such as oppression, deprivation, diversity and social change. The categorisation of social deprivation in the Indices of Deprivation, however, do not in themselves effect the social change necessary to address complex issues of a disadvantaged community, and the town where this study takes place remains in the political arena of regeneration funding through government institution intervention.

This social deprivation affects the personal identities of the women in the study in several ways. By 'belonging' to such a community and developing a personal place identity (Taylor, 2004) the women are embedded firmly in a community that is affected by social deprivation and, according to governmental departments, in need of social change. It is clear in the accounts that the women are affected by interactive social issues that contribute to social deprivation. The accounts are all health related and have contributed to the construction of health identity as part of lived experience. Therefore, the social deprivation present in this community affects the way that women construct their health identity.

The focus of this study on the health of perimenopausal women in this town has provided an opportunity to study the link between societal health and personal health. In this section, societal health in terms of a broad-based government ideology of what constitutes social deprivation is considered, as society has labelled this town a deprived community. The women's accounts to see how these personal accounts of health fit with societal aspects of social deprivation and found that a health-focused study additionally provides examples from everyday life of social deprivation. This suggests, as Sixsmith and Boneham (2003) theorise, that everyday community life provides a sense of identity within which health is a fragment, and that this is linked to and interactive with societal issues. Additionally, the ideological notion of regenerated community provided by government departments and aimed at addressing social deprivation has not filtered down in a positive sense into the everyday lives of the women. In 2000, the town was the 39th most deprived area of England and Wales; in 2004, four years into regeneration funding, the town was 38th most deprived area in England and Wales, falling further to 34th in 2007. The narrative accounts do not contain talk about improvements to community living or health or social change that has been affected in the area. Rather, they reflect the Indices of Deprivation in a negative sense, highlighting the problem more than the solution. This suggests that although they are interactive, there is conflict between the everyday experiences of the women and the ideological positioning of the government on social deprivation. The identity action of belonging to a community and explaining this in relation to health has highlighted this conflict.

The Indices of Deprivation give an overview of how society, in this case the government, tries to address social problems and social change. The broad-based categories prescribed by government as social indicators of all societal problems include health issues. The women's health narratives contained references to these same societal issues, as seen from a health perspective. In the accounts, the participants mentioned other aspects of societal health that affected them.

### *Everyday Identity – Two case studies of how identity construction in complex everyday situations*

This section considers two case studies from the research site that illustrate the complexities of real life identity and the levels of analysis available to understand how identities are constructed.

#### *Case study 1: Rene and Oldham family crisis group*

Although domestic violence is not framed in health terms in the institutional organisations of funding and management structures in Oldham, it inevitably impacts on the health of many women. National statistics show that one in four women will experience domestic violence in their lifetime. Considering the Indices of Deprivation, a woman who is experiencing domestic violence is also experiencing all seven of the prescribed domains of deprivation in addition to the personal and interpersonal oppression she is facing because of the situation she finds herself in. Oldham Family Crisis Group is a registered charity on Oldham that deals with aspects of domestic violence and forced marriage. The organisation celebrated its 30th anniversary in 2009 and continues to help women fleeing abuse in the home.

The group comprises of a women's refuge, a Zinda Dil refuge and second stage accommodation, outreach workers, counselling services and children's services and are administrated by office staff. The bed occupancy in the refuges are usually at capacity and demand for the service is high. However, in recent years and with funding changes, the future of the organisation is more uncertain. The ethos of the organisation is to put the women they help first the staff are proud of their caring and nurturing strategy and policy. However, due to funding demands they feel pressurised into using their resources on commissioning documents, audits and fulfilling the changing criteria that the local authority sets out for children's services. This political aspect of running a domestic violence refuge in a useful and meaningful way that respects the equality of the women users is an overriding factor in the future running of the organisation and provides a ready-made institutionalised conflict.

The women who use the refuges are varied in their personal situations. Many are fleeing their abuser with families, some are single women who are escaping forced marriage and some have multi-domain problems. This case study examines the identity construction of one of these women and attempts to understand how she is constructing her identity, including her health identity, on personal, interpersonal and institutionalised levels of analysis. The account was written on behalf of Rene, a lady who used the refuge service, by her refuge worker.

Rene was referred to the project and tenancy commenced soon after. She came through as a self-referral to the refuge and she was accepted as fleeing domestic violence – her abusers were reported to be her husband and her children. The abuse was physical from her husband and financial from all of them. When she first arrived she told staff that where she had been living people had kept smashing her windows and stealing from her. The refuge supported her as much as we could in the initial weeks after the referral but her over-riding mental health made it increasingly difficult and a referral to Zinda Dil (for women with possible mental health issues) was made.

She moved into sheltered accommodation in the year following.

Rene was born in India in 1939. Her mother died when she was young. After the death of her mother she was given the responsibility of caring for the family that consisted of her father and four brothers. At the age of 15 she had an arranged marriage to an older man. During this marriage she had a daughter and her husband was violent towards her. Her husband died and she returned to the family home because her in-laws declined for her to live with them as they believed she was a bad omen and she was responsible for the death of her husband.

Another marriage was arranged shortly afterwards and she had two children from this marriage. Both the babies died in the first year of their life due to neglect. Rene and her husband came to England and they had another two children. The marriage ended in divorce and her husband cited relationship difficulties, neglect of the children hoarding and bizarre ritualistic behaviours.

Rene moved out of the area and moved up and down the country securing short hold tenancies. Relatives had informed her that her children were settled in another town and she secured a tenancy with a Housing Association. Neighbours complained about her banging on the neighbours ceiling and keeping them awake. She was brought to the attention of Social Services when the Housing Officer visited the flat and they became concerned of her bizarre behaviour.

Later a visit was conducted by Social Services and they found that she did not sleep properly in a bed and dozed wherever she could. She had been hoarding rubbish and materials and had built a cave with these items. She kept the curtains closed as she did not like sunlight and would only venture out of her flat when it was dark. Due to her beliefs she had broken all light fittings, unscrewed door handles and she lived in the dark and used torches when required. The full extent of the house was crammed with items she had found. She had bought food in bulk which became out of date and stored cooked food in a way that was potentially hazardous. She declined to accept her pensions and benefits that were owed to her and it was unclear how she was receiving her money.

A social worker arranged for the flat to be cleared and she became angry with services and assaulted the social worker causing her serious injury. She was taken to hospital and detained under the Mental Health Act.

An assessment made by the psychiatrist described her as an odd lady. When she was admitted into hospital she was wearing 4–6 layers of clothing with two jackets. She had also taken two bags onto the ward full of DIY tools. Her explanation was that she needed these tools to repair and refit new locks . She believed that the electric vibrations from her home were being transferred to the ward, also the humming from electric wires were around her. She had no insight into her mental health difficulties and the problems her behaviour had caused because of her delusional ideas.

Rene was referred to the project soon after this. She settled down well in the local environment and began to engage with staff and other tenants. Her mood was much improved and she became more sociable with staff and began to engage with the support provided. She began to access services and during her stay staff supported her locate her children who were living nearby. Her children visited her regularly and the relationship developed. Feedback from other agencies was that she had improved her daily living skills and was engaging with services. She was diagnosed with schizophrenia and autistic spectrum disorder and was compliant with medication.

Rene was rehoused in warden controlled flat where she is currently living. She continued to receive support from the resettlement worker and then the outreach team. Rene occasionally visits the project and thank staff for the support that the organisation provided for her.

It is clear from this description of Rene's situation that there are complex personal, interpersonal and institutional issues at work in her life. Health issues play a predominant part in Rene's situation and her mental health issues remained undiagnosed for a long period of time. Her interaction with the domestic violence team at Oldham Family Crisis Group improved her situation and she received advocacy and mediation to help her negotiate her path to wellbeing. Rene's identity is clearly affected by her own personal health, her interpersonal relationships where she has experienced domestic violence and institutional aspects of how her situation is dealt with.

Therefore starting point for the study of Rene's identity construction is the personal, interpersonal and institutional aspects of her life. These would be the basis for any further studies into the way Rene has been affected, both positively and negatively, by the aspects above. The next step would be to match these aspects with appropriate identity actions. This process involves reading and rereading of Rene's personal account and identifying the movement of her identity on and axis of action rather than labelling individual situations. For example, Rene's tenancy with the domestic violence team clearly contributed to her feeling of belonging, as illustrated by her frequent visits and thanks to the staff. However, this identity action of belonging could so easily be translated into negative labelling should Rene be socially segregated as 'service user' or 'refugee'. It is important that the identity actions capture the flexible, flowing nature of identity construction so as not to trap the person inside a negative construction or stereotype.

It is clear from this overview of the identity construction of a victim of domestic violence both includes and extends the domains of deprivation and that health is a primary concern for these women and indeed the services. The usefulness of this modelling of identity construction in effecting social change in domestic violence provision is to highlight the issues of considering statistical information compared with the consideration of individual cases. Rene's case is an example of someone who has been assisted through the refuge to a more positive life, and is now experiencing fewer domains of deprivation. This schematically represented information within a valid model of identity construction could well influence the outcome of domestic violence funding on a societal level in addition to assisting the people involved in providing refuge to understand the issues Rene is experiencing, and their own reaction to it, and therefore reach out to her on an interpersonal level.

*Case study 2 – Everyday identity*

The second example of everyday lived experience and how the methodology could perhaps help women gain a voice is around the attitudes of women living in the research area regarding the way women should dress. This is an example of how identity and its construction affects everyday lived experience and how the word identity is used by women. Oldham is a cosmopolitan area where, following several years of racial disharmony, hard work has taken place to stop the social and cultural segregations mentioned in the Ritchie Report into Race Riots in (2001). Despite this work and marked improvement in race relations there are still emotive and contentious differences in the way that women's dress is regarded by some. Although this is often highlighted in the media and by various groups opposing opposite views, there is little recognition of these attitudes as dialectical opposites where both commonalities and differences can be understood on an axis.

Several perimenopausal women were interviewed and within their accounts gave their ideas regarding attitudes to appropriate dress. Below are excerpts from two of the accounts of these women.

Account 1. Shabnam is a 49 year old Asian woman living in Oldham with her three children and her husband. She works as a manger of a housing association and suffers from migraines on a weekly basis, diagnosed as stress migraines by her doctor.

> There are many issues that our communities are facing at the moment: high unemployment, people losing their homes and livelihood in the recession. But you know what most people go on about? What I'm wearing. I am a professional woman and I wear a burka. It's part of my identity. Am I subjugated? No. Do I wear this because I'm told to wear it? No. No one ever asks me why I wear it, they just assume. Plus they assume that the burka is only assigned to certain communities – many white women who have turned to Islam are also wearing the burka. Some women have gone a step further and are wearing the veil. If you

ask these ladies why, they will give you the same answer. We want to be judged on our personality and character. We want to retain our modesty. Is that a crime? It's wrong to judge. Leave me alone! It might not seem that this affects my health, but it does. I am subjected to bullying and hatred just because I stick to my own values. It makes me afraid. It really stresses me out. I'm going on the menopause and I don't want to be any more stressed out than I am. (Shabnam, Interview 1)

Account 2. Sharon is a 48 year old single mother of five. She lives alone and works in a nightclub at the weekend. Sharon had recently had an elective hysterectomy as her periods had become heavy and erratic. She is active in neighbourhood watch and is on her community management panel.

I hear about identity all the time. I'm really interested in it. For example, I would like to know just how the burka has become acceptable. People have their own opinions about burkas and Muslim women being repressed, I don't know if that's true or not. People from other cultures or religions or faiths or whatever won't get along if one faith sees itself as superior to others. Like making comments about girls wearing thongs openly or showing cleavage or a very short skirt. That's normal on my estate where I live and for other faiths to say it's wrong is backward and not an educated one. Why does everyone accept the burka but not the Hoodie? The hoodie conceals the identity of the person and so does the burka and the reason the people wearing hoodies are not allowed in shops is because it conceals their identity just like the burka does. Personally I am scared of women in burka cos I can't see their face. It makes me feel ill and anxious, you don't know what they are saying or doing. I'm forty eight years old and I don't. I'd be proud to go out dancing in a mini with a thong on. My boyfriend likes it and so do I. That's normal. I think that all identities in Britain today should be transparent and to not reveal your identity is being deliberately controversial. (Sharon, Interview 2)

By understanding these attitudes on a dialectical axis, equal weight is given to each cultural position. By comparing these two women's positions, a comparison of identity actions can perhaps be made and perhaps a better understanding of how these compare and contrast, of the commonalities and differences in the accounts. In terms of domains of deprivation, it is almost impossible to marry these two accounts to individual and prescribed singular domains, rather, and integrated approach where themes such as a common fear and common stress is an emergent and additional domain. So, again, these women's stories extend the domains of deprivation and present an opportunity to study how understanding and negotiation can be affected if the underlying reasons for the dialectical opposites are exposed.

In the next section, another way health is storied by society is examined. The media uses health as a vehicle to impact on the lives of women and gives another example of the fragmented, complex and unique ways in which the women use this consideration to construct the peri-menopausal health identity.

## Informing health – Mediated health in society

In order to take a critical approach to women's health, it is important to include external representations of health in society. The narrative accounts of the participants and field notes in this study highlighted the impact of the media on the health of the women. The media acts as a point of reference for the women in this study to construct ideological notions of health in the world. The women's accounts of peri-menopausal health suggest that when interpersonal relationships provide dissatisfactory health information, then the media is consulted. The analysis below reveals how the media operating in society is located in women's accounts of health.

Media representations of health are representative of institutionalised health in society and culture. Everyday talk in the initial meetings and the narrative accounts revealed the media as a situated point of reference for health matters and the participants' awareness of the media discourse. Therefore, a study of media representation of women's health is important because of the impact of these representations on the lived experience of women and consequently the construction of meaning through location of health understanding in media discourses. Lyons (2000) comments:

> The media play an important role in constructing identity through meanings that are embedded within dominant representations of health, health care, illness and disease. (Lyons, 2000, p.353)

To understand and interpret health identity construction in narrative accounts of the personal lived experience I have investigated representations that create meaning in the context of health. In the case of women's magazines, the professional and lay health advice (Kirkham, 2001) and vicarious experiences represented in the publications provide a health narrative which runs alongside the personal narrative. The participants revealed in the narrative accounts that the media played an important part in informing their health identity. Women's magazines were popular source of health information. Participants also mentioned newspapers, the internet, celebrity autobiography and television in the narrative accounts. In discussing the effects of the media on health, King and Watson (2005) suggest that:

> There has been relatively little so far that has attempted to bring together ideas about the ways in narratives of health and illness get shaped by, and echo in, various media genres (sometimes obviously, sometimes more subtly). (King and Watson, 2005, p.2)

In this section the interaction between the media as a societal tool and how this consideration affects the construction of health identity of perimenopausal women is discussed.

It is clear from the accounts that mediated health affected the women. All the women stated that they sought health information from different aspects of the media for different reasons. Only one of the participants said that she got her health information from leaflets or booklets from the NHS or her GP surgery and she explained that this was because she had previously worked as a receptionist in a surgery and was aware of this information from this experience. Most of the participants found their health information from women's magazines, newspapers, celebrity autobiographies, TV and the internet. This suggests that in seeking out this information all of the women in the study have been exposed to media health information. King and Watson's (2005) comment above about the way narratives are shaped by the media 'sometimes obviously, sometimes more subtly' (King and Watson, 2005, p.7) alludes to explicit material in the media sheltering below the institutionalised discourses of the grand narratives and discourses which compete for power and truth (Foucault, 1978) in society in influencing health identity. The provision of 'scientific facts and truths' in medically oriented discourse in the media is often contradictory from genre to genre. This provides hegemonic inequality (Gramsci, 1971) of power in media representations of health, disseminating conflicting information to recipients.

However, according to the 'uses and gratification' model of media theory, women often question this saturation of 'health truths' which objectify and oppress women, and seek out a more relational strand of media reporting which reflects their own style of narrative and consequently becomes more easily internalised into the health identity. This is supported by the emergent media themes in the narrative accounts. This section will look at the way that the women in the study have located media in their stories in order to link societal representation of health to the women's accounts.

### The media in women's everyday health talk

The narrative accounts revealed that the women located the media sources in their everyday story of health. The media was referred to from the first meeting through to the final debriefing. Most of the participants in this study were recruited through my advertisement in the media in a local newspaper. It is concluded from this and their participation in this study that these women were interested in health and were aware of the media. Additionally, the women often talked about the media in both their narrative accounts and in the initial and debriefing interviews. Some of the women mentioned health and the media in the contact phone call as they justified their interest in the study.

### Women's magazines: A multi-layered discourse of health

Most of the women in this study mentioned that they obtained health information from women's magazines. Many stated that they bought the magazines specifically for health information and tips, whilst some of the women said that they bought the magazine for other features but read health information by default. Katie spoke about her views on women's magazines:

> I buy women's magazines because I'm into health and I do I buy all sorts, buy the health ones for the tips, never used to buy them cos I thought Christians shouldn't be reading that crap, but I've got loads upstairs! You get good tips about eating or new things for skin. And there's tips and everything. I think most people do. Health touches everything. (Katie, Initial Interview)

Katie uses women's magazines for information about the health that she feels 'touches everything'. Whilst expressing an overarching narrative of how she feels she should fight information about health in this way as 'Christians shouldn't be reading that crap' and it goes against her spiritual beliefs, she values the information contained in the magazines in building her health and her changing perimenopausal health in terms of health tips. This implies that the women invest in the media model of health despite other ideological beliefs and are to some extent influenced by this.

### Daily newspapers: Overwhelming evidence of identity influence

Daily newspapers were recurrently mentioned in the narrative accounts. The participants initially read the papers for their news value, feeling that this was not the focus of the newspaper. Exceptionally, however, a major story about women's health presented in the newspapers was internalised by the women. Seventy-five per cent of the women in the study specifically mentioned 'The Menopause Test' feature. Linda had read the newspapers containing reports of this menopause test and had associated it with aspects of women's health in this study:

> Well there's this menopause test now that can tell you when it will, is likely to happen. It was in the papers, all the papers, I thought about this and you when I read it, I thought, 'I bet Jacqui has seen that!' Cos it's to do with this, isn't it...perimenopausal. (Linda, Study notes)

### Published autobiography – Identity by example

The women in this study talked about reading celebrity autobiography for inspiration. The general response was that these books which included the life stories of Victoria Wood, Jane Lapotaire, Helen Mirren and Angela Rippon, Ann Robinson and Ulrika Jonnson, were chosen originally for entertainment, but health information was gleaned from them and the life stories of these women detailing their health and social problems combined, motivated the women to get through their own problems. The women talked about these celebrity autobiographies mainly in the initial meeting. On review, this may have been prompted by the title of this study. This was helpful as the association between the format of these publications and what was required from the women in the study clarified many of the initial questions about the meaning of the study. All the women had read at least one celebrity autobiography and the most popularly read were Ann Robinson's 'Memoirs of an Unfit Mother' (60%) and Ulrika Johnson's 'Honest' (47%).

### The internet and women's health – If all else fails: Go online

Eighty per cent of the women in the study who were pre-menopausal and considered themselves to be on the menopause particularly found the internet useful for information about both women's health and general health. Carla typified the way the women spoke about the internet:

> Internet. I'm always sat at work on it. I don't like going to the GP because they're absolutely hopeless and whenever I go in for anything they just look at you as if to say, 'What's up with you?' I like the internet because you can look at things from all different angles, it's not the opinion of specific person is it. I like that. I look at things like cholesterol and hot flushes and mood swings. They can't know everything about everything, but you can find information about almost everything on the internet. (Carla, Interview 1)

Following on from the view expressed in the previous chapter's analysis by the women about mistrust and health providers, Carla explains the way that she salvages her narrative by consulting the internet for information she cannot obtain from her doctor. Like many women in the study, Carla explains that 'you can look at things from all angles' and consider the internet as providing a range of opinions and facts that are informative because 'you can find information about almost everything on the internet'. This popular view about the internet indicates that the women's relationship with the internet is important when gathering information to construct and reconstruct health identity.

## Television programmes – Comedy and the perimenopausal women

Several women said that women's problems got 'bad press' because of TV comedy. The TV show most mentioned was the Royle Family, a sitcom featuring a family from the North West of England (the choice of 17 women in the study). This TV series included an episode that dealt specifically with the menopause. In respect of this, Deborah, in her initial meeting mentioned the Royal Family:

> (Laughs) Oh yeah, the menopause, like Barbara in the Royal Family, when Jim finally makes a cup of tea! (Laughs). It's not funny really, it was a bit like my dad was with my mum when she was on the change. I know it's only on telly but it reminded me of that. Poor Barbara. (Deborah, Initial meeting – transcribed from field notes)

Deborah laughs along with her recollection of the TV show until she realises that it mirrors her parents' health experience during her mother's menopause, at which point she says, 'It's not funny really.' TV comedy is another example of the tone of discourse to switch attention away from the crisis in order to avoid the grand narrative. In this case, the dramatisation of Barbara's menopause in a comical way provides a gateway to understanding this crisis that many families face, as the viewers see the series as close to real life. Michelle was one of the women who mentioned the TV series Absolutely Fabulous in relation to women's health and the menopause:

> For me it was the funniest thing I have ever seen on Ab Fab when Patsy got osteoporosis and they thought they were on the menopause. They had a women's group and Eddie made them sit on plastic bags because of their pelvic floors (laughs). I hope I'm not like that, well I'm on it now, my periods are funny, but I don't have any bladder problems? Is that what happens? (Michelle, Initial meeting – transcribed from field notes)

Michelle again laughs at the comical representation of menopausal symptoms in Absolutely Fabulous, and has clearly internalised this representation as she suddenly and more seriously queries the possibility of developing the symptoms herself.

### Social media – Informing identity

The media operating in society is an area where health is strongly represented (King & Watson, 2005). The media has several obvious impacts on society and on identity construction through the presentation of information aimed at consumers in general, and often at specific consumers (Blumer & Katz, 1974). Due to the ever-increasing postmodern nature of lived experience the basic variety and availability of information due to the media has become a necessity of western society and women are major media consumers. Because of the growth of the media industry, the influence and dependency of society on the media changes society dramatically (Gergen, 1991).

Other than the obvious explicit impact of media on society, such as advertising and news media, there are more possibly fundamental effects of the media on health identity. Because of these more hidden impacts, such as political, social and culturally biased discourses (King & Watson, 2005) it is clear that the effect the media makes on society and identity is often more implicit than at first assumed. As the media construction of health is so powerful and reaches many areas of society (King & Watson, 2005), how the media affects women's health identity particularly in terms of the politics of women's bodies is investigated here.

## The connection between media and identity

> ...newspapers, magazines, and television provide a barrage of new criteria of self-evaluation. Is one sufficiently adventurous, clean, well-travelled, well read, low in cholesterol, slim, skilled in cooking, friendly, odour-free, coiffed, frugal, burglar-proof, family-oriented? The list is unending. (Gergen, 1991, p.76)

Gergen's comments above reflect the problems faced in everyday life when confronted by an unending media narrative. In early societies, social roles were defined largely by a social order based firmly in tradition (Giddens, 1991) and this would provide grand narratives in society by which people defined themselves. However, in society today there are so many roles available in the fragmented self that interaction with everyday life necessitates decision-making about how to construct identity. Giddens (1991) comments:

> What to do? How to act? Who to be? These are focal questions for everyone living in circumstances of late modernity – and ones which, on some level or another, all of us answer, either discursively or through day-to-day social behaviour. (Giddens, 1991, p.70)

The choices we make in society may be affected by tradition on one hand, and a sense of relative freedom on the other. Everyday choices about what to eat, what to wear, who to socialise with, are all decisions which position ourselves as one kind of person and not another. Giddens (1991) suggests that:

> The more post-traditional the settings in which an individual moves, the more lifestyle concerns the very core of self-identity, its making and remaking. (Giddens, 1991, p.81)

The media provides a route by which comparison of the self-identity and remaking of the self-identity is possible. Gergen (1991) suggests that the technology and in particular, the media, saturates the self with ever growing possibilities of identities presenting themselves. He comments that:

> Both the populating of the self and the multiphrenic condition are significant preludes to postmodern consciousness. To appreciate the

magnitude of cultural change, and its probable intensification, attention must be directed to the emerging technologies. (Gergen, 1991, p.49)

Gergen's 'populating of the self' and 'multiphrenic condition' return to the critique of the fixed identity. Gergen suggests that the fixed self is negated by the possibilities for many alternative roles within social interactions. Further, that as a result of taking up these multiple roles, the self is split into an array of self-investments in these roles. Goffman (1959) provides analysis of these role-playing selves in his dramaturgical theory. Goffman suggests that to keep order in society and the self, role-playing is a mediation of the two. This invites the critique that if the self is a collection of roles, with no real core, then there is no real 'self'. Role-playing is better described therefore as a 'best-fit' situation between the self and the social world. In terms of the health, the health identity is played out by necessity of the material self-embodied in the world by the discursive health identity.

### What the media means for health identity

Health is a concept that is of primary concern to the human situation. Our state of health, that is the physical state of our bodies, is a constant spatiotemporal consideration, and the way that we embody this in the world through our health behaviour is a signal to others as to how healthy we are. In turn, we internalise from available media representations of health, illness and wellbeing that impact on our own health identities. The media is particularly interested in women's bodies and attempts to control femininity in both positive and negative terms, as outlined below.

### Positive media health intervention

Many studies have been carried out focusing on how health is represented in the media (King & Watson, 2005). Fishbein and Yzer (2003) consider two models of designing health behaviour interventions. Fishbein and Yzer suggest that there are two approaches to health intervention design. The first, an integrated theory of behavioural prediction, proposes a bottom up design, where the person's current health beliefs determine the intervention, building on those aspects of health identity and modifying them through media representations. Conversely, media-priming theory proposes the introduction of new or alternative beliefs through the media, impacting on health identity and behaviour. Use of theory in media intervention suggests that what we perceive in the media is not solely for entertainment value, and is often motivated by different agencies and stakeholder for various reasons. An example of this is health promotion through the media.

Health policy such as healthy eating and health awareness is often disseminated through media sources such as advertisements and articles about positive health and strategies towards wellness. However, political aspects of health promotion, such as reports on government-sponsored studies like Societal Issues Research Centre (2001) discussed earlier, invite the critique that information about the negative aspects of health which may sometimes be withheld. In this case, the risks of taking HRT are selectively made available in this health intervention where the government wishes to promote the benefits of HRT.

**Negative media health intervention**

To make the media more accessible, different techniques are used to attract an audience. Media experts are aware that health issues concern the public in general and will often use stories about health to attract a larger viewing audience or readership. A negative consequence of this is moral panic (Mercer, 1990). By magnifying health issues, the media can influence other areas of society in social and economic ways. A health issue that has been extensively discussed on various levels is body image and the media. Thompson and Stice (2001) investigated thin-ideal internalisation and found that:

> Thin ideal internalisation is positively correlated with body image and eating disturbances. (Thompson & Stice, 2001, p.182)

This is an important area of research that investigates eating pathology which may eventually lead to death, and many studies (Hardin, 2003; Wilcox and Laird, 2000; Williams et al., 2003) have been carried out about the effects of the media on eating disturbances, particularly amongst women.

The examples above illustrate how the media is a tool for social representations of women's health and politicises women's bodies. The studies of anorexia show that women are influenced by body shape in the media and the government sponsored HRT reports in the media show the ability of the media to position women's bodies in society. This is not to suggest that women have no choice or discretion as to what media they decide to view; it was clear from the women's accounts that they had access to many forms of media. The saturation of society by the media, including media representations of women's bodies, impacts on the information available around women's health and influences identity through becoming institutionalised in everyday experience (Gergen, 1991). As can be seen above, women's everyday talk contains reference to media representations. The power dynamic of the media as an institution over individual women's experiences consequently creates inequality in society. Holding an ideological image of women's bodies directly affects not only health through issues such as anorexia and HRT, but also through objectification of women and their roles in society. This brings into focus the feminist standpoint as discussed in Chapter 4, where women aspire to freedom and valuing of difference within difference whilst the media produces representations in society which are implicitly political and influence women's health in a negative sense causing identity conflict. Therefore, the identity action of informing health through interaction with society through the media is problematic for the construction of health identity.

This conflict between personal everyday experience and ideologies provided by institutions in society was common in the narrative accounts. The women were aware of the media items they were exposed to, but not explicitly aware of the political and social mechanisms that drive such institutions as the media. In terms of this, the narrative accounts exposed influences from various areas of institutionalised power that, although the women were aware of the existence of a power dynamic, often framed this in terms of a crisis and became confused about the source of the power dynamic. This was illustrated in the narrative account by instances of images of situations where the power dynamic was clearly present in the narrative, but presented as mystical or perplexing to the participant as to who or what was responsible for their dissatisfaction. It is important to note that this dissatisfaction is at odds with the personal and interpersonal layer of women's health identity.

This conflict between personal everyday experience and ideologies provided by institutions in society was common in the narrative accounts. The women in this study often appeared satisfied with their own evaluation of who they are and how they relate to others in terms of health experience; the main dissatisfaction emerged through institutionalised health and the power and difference dynamics detailed in the positional and ideological layer of health identity as examined in this chapter. In many cases, the women found that they were resisting health in that they felt that their health experience was out of their control and that they did not have the power to move their narrative on to their satisfaction, causing crisis in health identity. In these cases there were no clear interpersonal images, but more feelings or instincts accompanied by metaphorical phrases in an attempt to explain how this dynamic was out of their control; in most cases the scenario was of 'us and them' with 'them' as a source of unidentified external control.

In the following section, implicit aspects of power and control that affect the fragmented perimenopausal health identity in terms of health services is considered. The ways that the women felt they were fighting for their health and the corresponding societal aspects of power involved in this experience are considered.

## Fighting for health – Us and them

Further to the above need for empowerment in voicing their attitudes and feelings about their health, the participants also talked about their experience of the medical model of health. In telling the story of their health, the women in the study described situations that they had encountered in various health situations that had impacted on their health identity.

These health situations were mostly facilitated by the National Health Service (NHS) as the main healthcare provider in the UK. None of the women in the study received private healthcare and all relied on the NHS as healthcare providers.

The NHS was set up in 1948 and is the largest organisation in the European community. Following a period of dysfunction on the 1990s, the NHS claims to be a patient-centred organisation that value their patients as equal partners to health professionals and encourage patients to make decisions and real choices about the NHS (NHS website, 2007). As primary and secondary care providers, the NHS operates a National Service Framework that aims to cover the highest priority conditions such as cancer and coronary heart disease. Additionally, the NHS undertook a full-scale modernisation program in 2000 from which emerged the NHS core principles. These include aims on a critical agenda such as valuing diversity of populations, responding to needs of individual patients, based on clinical need inability to pay, and reducing health inequalities.

The experiences of the women in this study did not always match these aims. Whilst some of these experiences were positive, many left the women battling institutionalised power and fighting for control of their own health. These difficult and challenging situations, which were often due to cultural, social or economic factors in the lived experiences of health in a disadvantaged community, were central to the salvage of many of the narratives (Frank, 2000a) and feature in all of the narrative accounts of health.

## The general practitioner

Some of the women in the study told stories of comfort and help received from their general practitioner. Those who were happy with their primary healthcare based this on a GP who listened to them and did not turn to alternative remedies for health solutions. Ruby explained how, during a visit to her doctor about abnormal cells or her cervix, she gained satisfactory information:

> So I got a bit upset and said I wanted to know more about it. He sat down and explained it to me for about half an hour and told me not to worry, it would get sorted out. I was upset but he was very nice and I believed him. At the end he gave me a fact sheet and I kept that so I could read off it to people who asked cos I couldn't remember what the doctor said cos I was so upset. (Ruby, Interview 1)

Katie also had a positive health experience with her doctor who she stated could be trusted implicitly. In instances where the participant was satisfied with the primary healthcare experience it was clear that the doctor or nurse involved had spent time explaining the nature of the health problem and provided enough information. Ruby does not need to search further than the interpersonal relationship for her health information, and therefore her narrative does not go on to the final layer of perimenopausal health identity, as there is no conflict. This suggests that the participant formed a good, communicative relationship with the healthcare provider and the narrative crisis was de-mystified by the provision of explanation and information. This supports the case for a relational model of health described in this book.

However, many of the women expressed dissatisfaction with their primary healthcarer. Using graphic imagery, they described difficult situations and the resulting distrust in the General Practitioner. Those women who were dissatisfied with primary healthcare often solved this problem by using other sources of information such as alternative health remedies or negative coping strategies that did not involve primary care providers.

Susan, for example, expressed frustration with her GP:

> No not at all. I think they was useless at the doctors erm but as I say on those couple of occasions where I do go, cos I don't like going to the doctors, but when I was going with headaches they started saying, 'Oooo how you feeling? And what about anti-depressants?' and I said, 'No I don't want to go down that road. No I don't feel

like I need to do that.' Erm so basically I think they are rubbish. Erm and not helpful at all. (Susan, Interview 1)

There was a clear mismatch between Susan's own evaluation of her health problem and the doctor's which raised trust issues between Susan and the medical model of health. As a consequence of these trust issues, Susan coped with her headaches by going to bed and not getting up until the headache had gone. Julie spoke about her GP in similar terms of 'they always fob you off.' Julie says that the doctors 'fob you off' where she means that they do not take her seriously or do not listen. Again, this raises trust issues and feelings that no matter what the health complaint, a wrong diagnosis will be made and that effort has to be made to get the correct attention and diffuse the perceived inequality. Yardley (1997) raises a valid point about the power relationships between doctors and patients. In a study about diagnosis of women's dizziness, she notes that:

> The dilemma faced by these women is whether to position themselves as a passive and defective body in the hands of doctors, or try to assert a more constructive role. (Yardley, 1997, p.117)

The accounts in this study reflect Yardley's findings that there is a dilemma to be faced by women in the healthcare encounter. In this study, an acute sense of frustration at the passive role the women felt they were adopting in this situation was evident, although this frustration was often not directed at the interpersonal healthcare encounter, but as a resistance to health in general. In extracts above, Julie and Susan are not speaking about their interpersonal relationship with their GP. It may be that they felt that their health experience (see Sixsmith & Boneham, 2003) are being ignored by health professionals, thus disempowering them in respect of and important aspect of their own experience. Whist describing a visit to the doctor, they do not use the singular 'he' or 'she' to describe and interpersonal encounter, but use 'they' to describe the collective dissatisfaction with their health experience. This suggests that in these cases, the voices of the ill person were not heard, often misdiagnosis occurred and the encounter was impersonal. Conversely, the women in the study felt that they deserved to have their voices heard in the medical encounter, and that to achieve this they had to fight for empowerment. This impacts on the fragmented health identity by embedding this feeling of disempowerment in the health experience and creating uncertainty and crisis in health encounters.

**The hospital ward**

The narratives of most of the women also contained strong images of dissatisfaction with hospitals. These were often associated with lack of consideration for individual needs by an unidentifiable person referred to as 'they' or 'them'. Often these images were associated with the removal of agency of the ill person, who turned into a 'patient' when entering the hospital ward. Colleen, who underwent a gastric investigation, felt that the process was impersonal and that she was objectified:

> I had to have erm a gastroscopy? And a colonoscopy without any aesthetic. And I've never had anything as bad, as frightening in my whole life. They don't warn you, oh you're just gonna get this and get that and you think yeah you can do that, it'll be alright yeah. Honestly, I felt like I was on a butcher's block. I felt as though I was....And it's terrible when you're awake. (Colleen, Interview 1)

Colleen's feeling about how she was treated was not directed at the doctors who performed the investigation. Colleen resists and fights for health on the ideological layer of the fragmented health identity. In the absence of control over what happened to her during the process and who was responsible for the lack of information communicated, Colleen again uses the collective 'they' when she described how she felt, using a strong metaphor of objectification; the 'butcher's block' representing the cutting up of a dead animal carcass.

This echoes McAdam's (1993) work on images and metaphors in identity construction, which suggests that the meaning-making process of images and metaphors underlines the parts of the fragmented identity for which adequate words cannot be found. Colleen clearly feels that her lack of control over her health situation caused her to form negative perceptions of the hospital ward. Lucy's experience of the hospital ward shows the transition from ill person to 'patient' and how Lucy felt the institutionalised power disregarded her person feeling's after an ectopic pregnancy:

> About another year after that I had an ectopic pregnancy. I wasn't psychologically damaged at the time but erm it was quite a complex thing to go through cos the operation is quite serious and stuff like that, it's quite frightening as well. Yeah but I find at the hospital nobody says anything to you, they put you on a ward with people that are having babies and people, all different gynaecological problems that they have. They put you on a mixed ward and for all they

> know you could be suffering psychologically. None of the nurses ever explained anything really, they were helpful but they didn't tell you anything about it. And also...Well they seemed very busy so, they seemed very busy a lot of the time so you don't think they are there to counsel you but you feel that they should be getting on with their work and you don't want to bother them. But no, nothing was really explained. Anyway.... (Lucy, Interview 1)

Again, the lack of interpersonal experiences on the hospital ward, in contrast to at home caused a health identity crisis for these women. The loss of agency through placement in a position where they are uncertain of what is happening to them impacts on their health identity, but, as Lucy points out, they do not feel that the hospital staff are to blame. Lucy links this episode of her story of building health to today by ending the narrative abruptly with an 'anyway', returning to the context of the present by asserting the she is strong. This indicates that this identity of strength that she used to fight her feelings that she was not understood are a thread that runs through the narrative account, and are reflected in the tone of the interview. The unequal power dynamic in this situation, with the hospital ward becoming an ultimate controlling influence in the outcome of the health crisis causes an external inequality, forcing the reconstruction of health identity from that of 'being a healthy person' to that of a 'patient identity', and further into crisis.

### The NHS as an institution

In some cases, dissatisfaction and anger was levelled at the NHS as an oppressive institution by disengaging from health professionals as people and engaging with the NHS as a disembodied and objectified institution. Linked to personal stories of health or the health of a loved one, the participants told how they had challenged the NHS as an institution even when they felt powerless to do so. Lisa took up the gauntlet of freedom and challenged the NHS when an alleged error caused her husband to die prematurely:

> Anyway I got there and he's died. As you can imagine, it was chaotic. But after I had sorted everything out and the funeral arrangements and stuff like that I got to thinking about things like this and I, I wondered why they didn't examine him. Because had they done they would have realised. He actually died with a pulmonary embolism and had they examined him they would have known, especially with the projectile vomiting, and er I got onto the ward manager by letter and

> pointed everything out to them. I did successfully sue them. I got some compensation. I said, 'I'm not actually blaming you for him dying but what I'm blaming you for is not carrying out a proper and appropriate examination. If you had have done you would have detected the problem and in the worst case scenario I would have at least been able to stay with him.' They may have prolonged his life for a few days or they may not but at least I would have been able to stay with him. He died on his own, you know. You get browbeaten. You see the thing is Jacqui I knew I were right. If I hadn't have known 100% I was right I wouldn't have pursued it, I would have made a fool of myself, but I knew I were right. I do know people who have had similar experiences and have thought, 'Oh well such a body's dead now.' And they think they can't do something like that, they think they can't battle against the forces, you know. I think there's a lot of it going on. (Lisa, Interview 1)

In this case, 'they' were the institution of the NHS. Lisa's battle with what seemed like disproportionate power that she describes as 'forces' embodies her stoical health identity which she empowers vicariously on her husband's behalf. This conflict in identity that Lisa is experiencing could be seen to echo by Frank (2000a) and Mishler's (1999) work which proposes that these kinds of conflicts create a crisis in identity. Lisa's ultimate belief that she deserved to be there when her husband died after nursing him through Parkinson's disease for 20 years empowered her to challenge the injustice she felt. In this way, she salvaged the narrative wreckage (Frank, 2000a) of an unending story and gained the closure that she felt was appropriate to her own needs in this situation. Lisa did not allow her positional and situational health identity to oppress her and continued to 'battle against the forces' for her personal freedom, preferring to believe in her own narrative of 'I knew I was right'. Cynthia sums up the feelings of many of the participants in her confusion about who is responsible for the confusion about who 'they' are. Cynthia's health ideology is heavily invested in the financial aspect of health. Her original dissatisfaction with the NHS and what she feels is an impersonal service extends to the fact that she feels like she is paying for something she is not satisfied with but has no power to object. Cynthia feels that the only currency of freedom from the oppressive system is financial. Her image of Spain as a health utopia reflects her awareness of her ageing body and the eventual need for medical attention which she feels is impossible in her current situation because of accumulated bad experience with healthcare provision in her existing position. In examining who is responsible for this situation, Cynthia asserts that it is not the fault of the doctors, but is unsure as to whether the NHS or the government, or both, are responsible.

### Oppression and the health situation

The patriarchal nature of medicalised health was present in the narrative account in the form of stories about mistreatment in hospitals. The women gave accounts of perceived bullying in images that highlighted the fact that although the women knew that this was wrong, they were unsure of who to blame. An example of this is Sarah's story about childbirth, when an authoritative discourse, in the guise of rules issued by staff, became confusing as it contradicted the instinctive interpersonal nature of the health situation.

> When I was bathing her once, in a separate bathroom, I was washing her and when I was going I heard a voice saying 'Don't go!' I couldn't see anybody. I said 'Is there anybody there?' and this voice said 'I'm here!' There was a woman behind the screen and I asked her what she was doing there. I got into trouble for that actually, the breast feeding sister said, 'Mrs Anderson, you mustn't carry your child around.' But she was mine. They didn't really like me helping this woman, I don't know why, but I don't think it was because I was helping her, I think it was because I was doing something of our own. (Sarah, Interview 1)

This suggests that although the women were aware that they were dissatisfied with their objectification and the hegemonic attitudes they perceived, they regarded the National Health Service as a power which could not be defeated without either great effort or taking the risk of going to unqualified sources for treatment. Kath's narrative (as outlined in Chapter 6) explains that she had to resort to an illegal abortion because of several oppressive factors. This constant reconstruction of health identity in terms of 'us and them' power dynamics places the women in this study in a privileged standpoint (Harding, 1996; Harstock, 1999), that of being able to peruse the power dynamic that they are dealing with and critique it using values of difference within difference. For example, Caroline in Chapter 6, recognised the lack of 'taken for granted' health and social milestones in her life due to her sexuality. Holly, in the same section, acknowledges that this lack of health information, which other people have access to, makes her future health identity open to uncertainty.

This is characteristic of feminist standpoint theory (Harding, 1996; Harstock, 1998) which has been criticised for generalising across class and culture and not valuing the individual situation and position of individual women. In this case, however, Caroline and Holly, (who are able to survey the health milestones for women, both social and physical) have reflected on their health lives and each identified an area, which they perceive as 'different' to other women and in crisis. This had led them to a unique standpoint from which they can critique aspects of the world that are available to other women, but not to them, therefore causing inequality. This is expressed in this study by the explanations of gay women of their sexuality, whereas none of the straight women in the study mentioned or explained sexuality, suggesting that without the standpoint of perceived difference, sexuality for them, was taken for granted.

The analysis of women's personal, interpersonal and societal experiences and consideration of health has shown that on all these levels women are concerned about their healthcare services. Issues around GP care, hospital care and medical issues in general are prominent in all the accounts and conflicts occur on a level where women cannot understand why they are treated in an unsatisfactory way. As discussed earlier, health is a gendered concept and women's bodies are politicised in many ways. These include the ability of women to carry out roles in society around the reproductive cycle, and the medicalisation of women's' bodies around the reproductive cycle. The objectification of women is also centred around dualist concepts of milestones such as menstruation and menopause. The women in this study have reacted to this institutionalised hegemonic politic by explaining their dissatisfaction with the National Health Service as an ideology of health in society. The women's accounts do not explicitly accuse or blame the NHS, but hold more of a disappointed tone that their expectations of the National Health Service have been thwarted. This is closely linked to the positioned and situated deprived community that the women live in. In terms of health, deprivation includes deprivation of health facilities in this community that in turn encourages health inequalities, particularly amongst low-income groups such as single parents and disabled people. Therefore, coupled with the NHS that is a patriarchal institution that often objectifies women, the participants in this study also contend with a broad-based deprivation on a social level that includes health services. The reaction from the women in this conflict of ideological expectations and everyday experience is that of resilience and stoicism and implied feminism in the form of taking on an institutionalised power to combat social inequality.

Even so, the expression of this implicit feminist action was problematic for the women. Stated previously in this analysis, none of the women stated that they were feminist or indicated that they had any knowledge of feminist theory. Consequently, the narrative accounts were based on the women's dissatisfaction with patriarchal institutionalised power dynamics and the difficulties faced by the women who felt that they needed to challenge these in some way. The women saw this study as a definite route for action, and at the initial meetings almost all the women expressed the need to 'get my story out' (Kath) and 'tell someone who will listen' (Cynthia) about their health experiences. This illustrates the need for research to include these voices and, taking into account the amount of research the women performed into their own health experience in order to be able to tell their story, the level of expertise the women, as experiences of health, bring to the research arena.

These accounts reinforce the importance placed on the medical discourse of health as illustrated earlier and provide an explanation of the power dynamics, which force the medical narrative into crisis, causing the search for knowledge to divert to other competing truths about health for a solution. In the light of this dissatisfaction with the medical model of health due to the uncertain nature of who is to blame for discontent and confusion, and consequent loss of agency of personal health, health often becomes mystified. In this situation, the participants often explained their health in terms of spirituality.

## Controlling health – If I am good then I will be well, that is what I believe

The theme of control over one's own health is continued here with spirituality. Murray and Zentner (1989) have formed a definition of spirituality that has been adopted for inclusiveness within healthcare settings as follows:

> ...a quality that goes beyond religious affiliation that strives for inspiration, reverence, awe, meaning and purpose, even in those who do not believe in any good. The spiritual dimension tries to be in harmony with the universe, strives for answers about the infinite, and comes essentially into focus in times of emotional stress, physical (and mental) illness, loss, bereavement and death. (Murray & Zentner, 1989, p.259)

This definition aims at inclusiveness for not just religious spirituality but also non-religious spirituality. The definition was developed in order that healthcare professionals would be aware of and respect the spiritual needs of patients. Ross (2006) considers the awareness of the spiritual needs of the patients in healthcare a relatively new concern and Swinton (2006) recognises that spirituality is part of a fragmented identity and that a sense of spiritual identity should be recognised in care giving settings.

Spirituality, then, is distinct from religion as according to Murray and Zentner (1989) it includes non-religious thinking. Martsolf and Mickley (1998) discuss spirituality as a collection of meaning, values, beliefs and a sense of connection that may or may not include a higher being. On a societal level, spirituality is often present in organised or non-organised religion where groups of people gather to follow an example given by a higher being. This is usually represented in terms of guidance towards goodness and away from evil. Organised religion, in the view of some people, can be political and powerful. Wright (2005) reflects on spirituality and health and warns that spirituality can:

> ...become a business, a vehicle for control. (Wright, 2005, p.202)

Wright draws together the complex relationship between the responsibility of health professionals to the people they care for and the organisations they work for. He comments that health policy-making has recently required healthcare workers to attend to the spiritual needs of their patients as well as their own. This suggests that, at the level of society and organsational ideology, guidelines are in place for the spiritual care of individuals under the care of the NHS. The following section takes excerpts from the accounts of some of the women in this study and examines how spirituality affects their health experience.

Many of the narratives were about how the participants believed a divine power was at least partially responsible for their health status, or had some effect on this. Ramondetta and Sills (2004) suggest that various kinds of coping strategies are employed in the health experience:

> some develop a collaborative coping style that involves what patients describe as an active exchange with their God, others approach decision making more passively using their spirituality to defer making choices and there are those who see themselves as self-directed problem solvers. (Ramondetta & Sills, 2004, p.183)

This lack of power over the personal health situation is closely linked to the powerlessness felt in their relationship with institutionalised health, for example, on admittance to hospitals for the women. It is also linked to their political relationship with their deprived lived experience. Handing over power to a higher force or indeed assigning responsibility for health to an all-encompassing power was a coping strategy used by many of the women in the absence of confidence in the medical model of health.

**If I am good...**

Some of the women in the study spoke of belief about health encompassing the concept of religious behaviour. Holly discussed her health beliefs regarding her depression in terms of her behaviour as a good Christian:

> I mean there have been times when I have been through depression I felt as if that area of my life had failed and it was almost as though, you know, you can't have enough faith. For you to get in that sort of state. That was the initial thing that made me feel worse for a bit. Yeah. And erm I didn't blame God either because I thought he's not bound to heal me on request you know it wasn't him who brought illness and sickness into the world it was the devil. You know he made a perfect world and it got made corrupt and messed up so I didn't turn round and blame him either but instead I looked to him and trusted him that he could put me right and heal me you know. But in the meantime I needed to look after myself. And have the right attitude and approach about it. (Holly, Interview 1)

Holly speaks about failure in terms of her health identity, as she had not managed to control her depression and links this closely with her lack of faith. She also lays blame on the devil for bringing illness and sickness into the world. Holly's faith provides her with a facility to relinquish personal responsibility for her illness on one hand, by laying the blame for it on the devil, and feels that, on the other hand, God should be able to cure her, if only she had enough faith. McAdams (1993) explains that aspects of faith in identity are important meaning-making aspects of life, and help to bring order to chaotic narratives. In this study, many stories were told of faith in conjunction with critical illness and the dynamics around this which brought meaning outside the medical model of health to illness. This complex interaction of failure, blame, and faith are all fragments of the health identity that are used to attempt to control illnesses which are perceived as out of control and create a narrative crisis.

None of the narrative accounts mentioned individual spirituality in terms of healthcare in the NHS even though many of the women had received hospital in-patient and outpatient treatment. This suggests that although the ideological aims of NHS policy-making are in place (Wright, 2005) the women in this study still found that they had to look elsewhere in their individual spiritual experience for guidance.

Cindy also spoke about her belief in God influencing health. When Cindy's daughter's injured leg could not be diagnosed by the hospital, Cindy asked 'Why God couldn't you heal her'. Cindy speaks about the story of her daughter's injured leg in close conjunction with their shared faith. Again, Cindy expresses her need to control the healing of her daughter's leg and queries the act of prayer in terms of healing. Control is therefore handed over to God for the healing of her daughter's leg, and whilst she asks God why He can't heal it now, she also asserts her faith that, in time, that he will heal the leg. In a similar circumstance to Holly, the lack of control over the healing process or cure is given over to a perceived higher being who will, in time, salvage the crisis in the illness narrative (Frank, 2000a).

This suggests that the crisis of narrative in conjunction to handing control over to a higher being negates the possibility of personal responsibility and agency in the health identity and provides an alternative meaning-making process for pain and suffering outside the institutionalised healthcare. For Cindy, Holly, and many other women in the study, this spirituality narrative is an enduring thread running through the health identity and an important factor in the construction of the perimenopausal health identity when the changing self is often in crisis. In these terms, spirituality is not directly linked to the health experience in society through healthcare and health relationships with others, but embedded in the personal identity and expressed as an alternative source of pastoral care, separate from the 'spirituality in healthcare' agenda of the NHS.

## Acceptance of health problems through understanding spirituality

Caroline, who is a Buddhist, speaks about how personal awareness promotes a feeling of agency in her health identity. She explains how Buddhism has helped her reach a stage where she has an acceptance of her ill health that promotes a more holistic view of health:

> So I think Buddhism has made me more aware of myself in my body because I meditate, you definitely can't meditate, you can't only do things with your head, you have to relax and bring your attention

> to your whole self. If you do meditate only with your head you end up a big space and it's not very balanced and it's not very good for you. Also the other thing that Buddhism teaches us is that everything is impermanent including the body so when something goes wrong, that's normal. You know, so you don't go, 'Oh my goodness, I'm developing a knee problem' you think, 'Well. I'm 40 it's incredible that my knees have lasted that long.' My body is impermanent, its normal for bit of it to go wrong, and it also teaches that life is not satisfactory. So Buddhism treats the mind and the attitudes not the condition. So you can have two people with cancer and one can just be ridden with hatred and injustice and you can have somebody else Buddhist or not who says, 'Well, cancer happens, why not me?' Is a much more intelligent question, I'm not so special. (Caroline, Interview 1)

Caroline's narrative suggests that she understands how health identity is related to, but not constituted by, material illness. This is important in the context of Caroline's perimenopausal identity, as she has reached a point at the time of the narrative of acceptance and no longer feels the need to control her health. Caroline's holistic awareness of how the mind and body are connected and acceptance of the impermanence of the body is interesting as it negates the urge to look for a cure for illness. This acceptance of the condition brings the realisation that, whilst medicine is available and some illness can be cured, the amount of psychological suffering is proportional to the amount of control over the attitude to illness. This more holistic coping strategy infers a more positive internalisation into the health identity and allows for the reconstruction of health identity in terms which acknowledge both the body as fallible and the social world as a place where the embodiment of the fallible body reduces the narrative wreckage caused by illness. Consequently, the salvage of the narrative (Frank, 2000a) and reconstruction of health identity require understanding and awareness of the inner self with less reliance on the external world and institutional power dynamics. However, as Caroline points out, this coping strategy requires time, attention, and self-discipline and, in the western world, is not accepted as 'the norm'. Again, Caroline's reliance on her individual spirituality as a coping strategy reflects the way that the women in this study have separated their spirituality from healthcare but aligned it with health.

### Mind, body and spirit

Similarly, the holistic health discourse of, as the participants often described, 'mind, body and spirit' is not widely accepted as an institutionalised grand narrative. Many of the women in the study made strong statements about holistic health. Pat commented that:

> Its really important to me, definitely, cos its mind, body and spirit. It's not separate, but all one. They are separate, but all one. And if I can't have that I can really feel it, me. It's like I'm somewhere else. Things start to come through, intuitive things in my dreams as well, quite strong and that's when I know things are wrong and I need to eat more healthily. I need to take time for myself. I feel like my feet are not on the ground, I'm off balance. I think if I didn't have that my life would be a lot more chaotic. (Pat, Interview 1)

This suggests that Pat's health identity, the way she feels about her healthy self, is constantly in a state of flux. Pat's awareness of this, however, enables her to have some control over her health identity and how she feels by regrounding herself. Within Pat's fragmented health identity the need to balance and control her health is important in ordering her health identity. Pat refers to balance many times in her narrative account, and many of the women in the study use the words 'balance grounded' when discussing health beliefs and the metaphor of 'feet on the ground' when talking about strategising for health. This suggests that the personal monitoring of health and the need for a health balance towards wellbeing on the illness/wellbeing scale are of paramount importance to the women in the study, and to obtain this balance they often look to a higher force to help them control their health. Again, Caroline's and Pat's reliance on their individual spirituality as a coping strategy reflects the way that the women in this study have separated their spirituality from healthcare but aligned it with health. As mentioned earlier, many of the participants mistrusted the healthcare providers and found conflict between lived health experience and the ideological notions and hegemonic practices they perceive as present in the NHS. This conflict left many of the women powerless in their fight with what they considered to be a force they were fighting against. The effect of the media on the health of the women in this study leaves them saturated in a sea of health information that they are powerless to control. In addition to this, the effects of living in a disadvantaged and deprived community have impacted on the lived health experience of these women both implicitly and explicitly in a political sense. Although they have a strong sense of place identity and the identity action of belonging is powerful for the women, their location and positioning in society is deprived and impacts on their health, possibly outside their awareness. The combination of these on the women's health experiences must be daunting and perhaps the women in this study have found comfort in looking to their individual spirituality as a reliable source of non-political pastoral care. None of the women in the study referred specifically to organised religion of the kind Wright refers to as 'a vehicle for control.' Rather they are looking to an individual sense of wellbeing and a relationship with their own spirituality outside the politicised health arena.

The control of health through spirituality, then, whether it be by sharing the responsibility with a perceived higher force, taking personal responsibility for that control, providing meaning-making outside the social ideologies of institutionalised health, or balancing these three, is important to the women in this study. This supports Ramondetta and Sills (2004) findings.

## Returning to past health experiences – Back to the future

The images around family life and the structure of the family in the narrative accounts were an important factor in contributing not only to the past and present representations of health, but also future health ideology.

### Family structures and health

Many of the women in this study were single parents and felt that this and its stigmatisation in society affected their health. Julie comments on how life as a single parent, which reflects Popay's (1992) work on women's tiredness, affects her work/life balance and made her ill:

> But I think I had got shingles because I was that run down, you know I mean that's what I said to me mum, when I finished at Lewis', I said 'I'm not working full time again with being on my own with Sam.' Cos I was just knackered. Its not that I don't want them to think bad of me its more of a case of, I want to look as though I'm coping. Everyone says single parents can't cope, and in some ways I don't cope that well, I get run down and ill with work and all that, but I like to look like I am. Its like to me, if I've got a load of ironing, like I have, in the back room, and me mum comes up she goes, 'Have you not done your ironing?' I go, 'No, I just iron it when I need it!' then she thinks its cos I'm on me own, but it's just cos I don't want to be up half the night and ill next day! (laughs). (Julie, Interview 1)

Julie's desire to 'look as though I am coping' links to the interpersonal layer of the fragmented health identity in the previous chapter where coping and performing a family role are aspects of the relational health identity. Julie's position as a single parent and her struggle with this makes her want to appear that she is coping in performing her role as a parent in what is often seen as different to and lesser than (Sixsmith & Boneham, 2003) the patriarchal family structure (Coser, 1977). In addition to this, Julie is fighting to keep healthy, which links to another key aspect of the ideological health layer. Julie's position in society as a single parent is clearly causing conflict in her fragmented health identity. This positioning in society, which conflicts with traditional family structures, causes a social inequity and is a concern of critical theorists such as Prilleltensky (2005). Prilleltensky's critical approach to complex social problems such as single parenthood being seen as a lesser family structure than a heterosexual two parent family structure recommend interventions towards wellbeing. In Julie's case, 'looking like I am coping' to other people highlights her isolation and sense of social injustice at her perceptions of society's view of single parents. Intervention, for Julie, would provide a support structure that is lacking in her narrative accounts and, according to work on social capital and support systems in deprived areas (see Boneham & Sixsmith, 2003) improve Julie's wellbeing and perception of coping.

Two of the women in the study were lesbian and told how their sexuality impacted on how their family life in many ways with a knock on effect for their health status. Kay spoke about her fractured relationship with her son and how she felt this made her ill:

> My dad accepted it (sexuality) right away but my mum was devastated for six weeks. We did see each other and we kept crying every time we saw each other but now she's absolutely right as rain. And she's really supportive and everything and more supportive with Andrew (son) now that what she ever was. Since I came out, but that's because what he's been through. Because of me being gay. Its heart breaking knowing, it's awful knowing what I've inflicted on Andrew. I could just cry every day over what I've inflicted on him. It's made me depressed. (Kay, Interview 1)

Kay comments that the effects her sexuality have had on her family life have made her depressed and in turn impacted on her perimenopausal identity by causing a conflict between her becoming, building and changing health and controlling aspects of societal family structures of health that imply how her life trajectory 'should' progress within her interpersonal relationships.

Women in the study who were part of a traditional family structure at the time of the narrative account protected their position fiercely, claiming that this improved their wellbeing. Colleen, whose first marriage was abusive, became depressed because of the dynamic of this relationship and the low self-esteem she was experiencing. However, she describes her current relationship as more positive and says that it has helped to reconstruct a positive perimenopausal health identity:

> Yeah and he (husband) went to live with his mum and that was the end and then filed for a two year separation, but I must say within a couple of months – well I wasn't interested in men – but within three weeks I'd met the person I'm married to now. He'd asked me to go out with him and I did go out with him but I found him very young. He is younger than I am and I did think he's too young for me and I wasn't very interested in men but he hung there and hung in and I ended up marrying him in 82. So I hung in a few years and then we got married in 1982. And Catherine was born in 1983. So she was born and I've had a very happy life since then. My present husband has built up my self esteem and just that has made me more healthy and look forward to life and look after myself. (Colleen, Interview 1)

Single women in the study, though highlighting less time constraints on their health solutions, expressed their wishes to be part of a family unit, usually citing their hope of having children to improve their wellbeing and progress through women's health milestones in the correct order as the reasons for this. Pat's explanation of this was typical of the younger single women in the study:

> When I was younger I never really ate properly and was using substances, but now I have more awareness and insight into myself for example, I need to... I can't do this, and I would be a lot healthier. A lot of it is to do with my future plans for getting married and having kids, to keep my body healthy for future children are more important and I'm building it up for that. Getting more healthy and fit for future children. (Pat, Interview 1)

Here Pat returns to her childhood and adolescent health situation to reinforce how she is building her health. Although she considers herself perimenopausal now at age 35, Pat still makes future plans for building her family, returning to past health to qualify this. Returning to previous constructions of health was central in constructing future health and this will be examined more closely in the next section.

## Family health behaviour and its impact on perceived future health

As observed in Chapter 6 the interpersonal relationships in the family of the participant often had an impact on the present and future health ideologies. However, the differences between the patriarchal hierarchical family structure of the Weberian ideological model of the family based on hierarchical power (Coser, 1977) clearly clashed with the more postmodern Foucaldian (Foucault, 1978) ideological model of the postmodern concept of family today. Many of the women had grown up in families where the father was the head of the household, and finding themselves in a situation other than this had various implications on their expectations of their future health. In many cases, they had adapted their parent's health behaviour to better fit the model of wellbeing mediated to them in the present and projected this into their future health, comparing it to the outcome of their parent's health situation. Brenda spoke about how caring for her father and mother through their illnesses had formed an expectation in her that she would be looked after by her children when she was older:

> Because I looked after my mum and dad when they were ill, I still look after my mum now really, even though she's in a home. But we were a proper family with no divorce. Now I've had a divorce and I'm married to someone else I suppose my children won't be like me, running round to look after me when I'm old and ill. Its not the same these days, I wouldn't expect it I suppose, well I would but I suppose it would be better if I went in a home as well when I'm like that. They're too busy. (Brenda, Interview 2)

Brenda felt duty bound to care for her father and has lived with the guilt of putting her mother in a home as it disobeyed her father's dying wish to her to care for her seriously ill mother, (who needed 24 hour care) at home. Brenda has observed the change in family structures through her life by returning to familiar health situations and comparing them to her health experience today. She concludes from this returning that she does not feel that the same level of commitment towards caring for other family members is present in her family today. Brenda hints that this is a result of her remarrying and losing the traditional patriarchal control of the family. This reflects Foucault's (1978) changing model of the family and how responsibility is perceived and disseminated more lightly than in the Weberian model, thus deflecting responsibility for health onto health institutions.

## Societal health – The impact of narrated positional, situated and ideological health representation

In this chapter, aspects of positional, situational and ideological representation of health in society in terms of how the women in this study experienced them have been examined. The identity action of belonging is explained in the light of the women in this study living in a deprived community. The indices by which this deprived community are measured is a societal construction of positioning and location in society. This forms a layer of societal health which lies above the lived experience of individual health and related health. Within this layer of societal health, it was found that the women also expressed their conflict with institutionalised health in society through aspects of media, healthcare and the NHS in particular, spirituality and family structures. All these aspects of societal concern are interactive and independent of the indices of deprivation measurement. In addition to this, the conflict that the women experienced in relation to this societal experience of health fall within the remit of a critical health agenda for social change (Marks et al., 2001; Prilleltensky & Fox, 1997). By studying health in the context of society, culture, politics, ideology, spirituality and personal experience an understanding of how the women have constructed their perimenopausal health identity is attempted in the light of personal, interpersonal and societal considerations. In this chapter the movement to the societal layer of identity actions, the health focus appears to have moved from reproductive health to generalised health in the context of living in the world for the women in this study and this is shown in Figure 8.1. In concluding this chapter, it is important to point to the layered theorising of the previous analysis of chapters. In these terms, Chapters 6, 7 and 8 overlay each other in that they are all emergent from the same accounts, but have been deconstructed according to the personal, interpersonal and societal representations of health present in the accounts. Therefore, Chapter 8 overlays the personal and interpersonal accounts of health and provides a health landscape on which the women position their lived experience of health. In these terms, the previous chapters are inclusive of the personal and interpersonal accounts and provide a context for these.

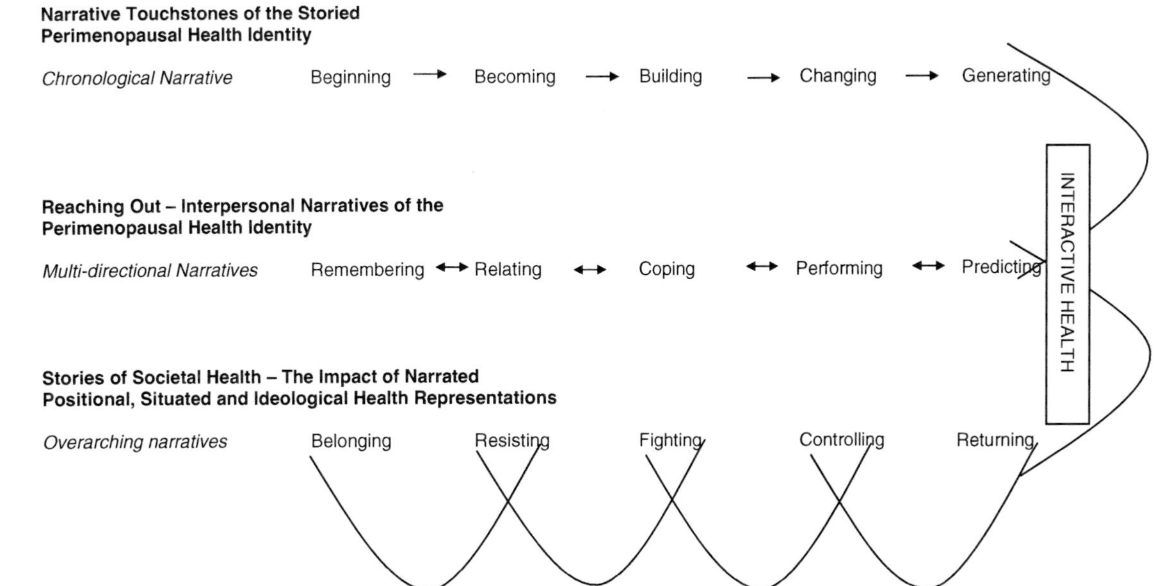


*Figure 8.1* Women's health identity actions – Personal, interpersonal and institutionalised health

# Part III

# Praxis

So far this book has covered theory and voice, bringing together the lives of women overlaid onto a theoretical landscape. Remembering the critique of theory and the suspicion regarding validity of qualitative research, it is often difficult to convince those who are tantalised by statistics that there is a 'real life' application of critical theory in the 'real world'.

This final chapter brings theory to praxis as consideration is given to how the model that emerges completes the bridge from identity as an idea to how identity construction works in practice. The emergent model is explained in terms of the existing everyday lives of women who experience identity construction.

# 9
# Identity Actions: Bringing about Social Change

It has been shown in this book that women construct their health identity throughout their whole life using medical milestones of women's health and social experiences of health as chronological touchstones and markers of meaning-making. The personal monitoring of the holistic health status in the narrative accounts has been integrated with interpersonal experiences of health, and embodiment of health identity in society, to theorise the construction of a health identity that included the possibility of fluidity and flexibility in the light of both illness and wellbeing.

Analysis of the women's narrative accounts of their health life stories revealed two main narratives on which the women based their health story; the medical narrative and the relational narrative. McAdams (1993) argues that the life story constitutes identity:

> Identity is something of collaboration between the person and the social world. The two are together responsible for the life story. (McAdams, 1993, p.93)

The women who took part revealed their health identity by giving medical and relational accounts of their identity and identity construction through the lifespan, culminating at the perimenopause. By combining the personal, interpersonal, situational and positional levels of analysis (Murray, 2000), these two strands of narrative used by the women in the accounts exposed problematic areas for the reconstruction of the mid-life health identity. The relational narrative strand exposed a smooth flow of explanation with a family-based, multidirectional timeline taking in past, present and future representations of health. This narrative provided little problem for the women in the study when faced with a health crisis, as they were able to draw on close interpersonal relationships in order to salvage the narrative account (Frank, 2000a). However, the medical narrative was more problematic. The relational and medical narratives were tightly interwoven in the accounts, and problems were exposed when the women attempted to apply an interpersonal relational narrative to a crisis that involved institutionalised health. The effects of institutionalised health, which were not explicitly stated in the accounts, were revealed through the examination of images and themes in the narrative accounts relating to the social location and positioning of the participants, institutionalised healthcare, feminist action and mediated health. The implications for these personal, interpersonal and institutionalised health effects and the perimenopausal health identity further below in terms of an interactive model of health identity.

## How the story ends

This book began by introducing the current progress of health psychology and research into women's health in terms of the power dynamics between the health professionals and lived experiences of women's health. In these terms, it was concluded that whilst women's health identity has been investigated in the context of the medical setting, little research has been conducted from a critical, person-centred position. Also, that this critical, person-centred position was necessary in order to elucidate the construction and reconstruction of women's health identity in order to relate theory to praxis in intervention, turning the focus from the 'patient' in medical terms to the person who is experiencing health on an axis of illness and wellbeing. Further, the objectification of women and the enduring Cartesian dualist (Descartes, 1647, in 1969 translation) paradigm of the medical model of health have limited the nature of research into this important area of health psychology. This work, therefore, has addressed this gap in knowledge of the process of construction of women's health identity from a person-centred perspective by studying the narrative accounts of perimenopausal women in order to investigate how the personal health identity is constructed and reconstructed during health milestones throughout women's lives up to the perimenopause. In order to do this, the process of identity construction on personal, interpersonal and ideological levels (Murray, 2000) combined with a methodological narrative model of tones, themes and images were combined to analyse the accounts of women who took part in the study, forming a multidimensional account of their health identity.

## Monitoring health

The process of consideration and embodiment of health experiences in the construction of health identity is expressed in this study through the women's constant monitoring of health. The participants tracked their health through personal, interpersonal, ideological and positional levels of analysis (Murray, 2000), showing that the monitoring of their physiological and psychological health status is a holistic process. An example of this is Holly's personal assessment of her pre-menstrual tension as part of her reproductive health, its devastating impact on her personal relationships and her consequent treatment by the institutionalised health system. This holistic assessment of the health experience surpasses the portrayal of health psychology in the literature review in the introduction of this thesis, exposing a gap in knowledge that highlights the importance of the consideration of the holistic nature of health identity outside the Cartesian dualistic model of health. This process compares with Bhaskar's (1978) model of critical realism where the intransive realism of the physiological body is linked to identity construction through the transive relativism of the health experience in the social world. Generative mechanisms, underpinning the interactions of these to form the health identity are represented in this study by this holistic monitoring of the health status.

## Institutionalised health and institutionalised feminism – A dialectical explanation

When considering their relationship with health, the women explained their experiences through vivid imagery. Whilst none of the women stated that they were feminists, their pro-choice stance on abortion and other interventions into their fertility might suggest that they were in fact informed feminists. However, control of pregnancy and fertility in this study was often seen as a desperate measure, dictated by cultural and economic position and situation of these women. The narrative accounts contained sub-narratives that revealed descriptions of identity in crisis surrounding fertility, such as Louise's confusion about sterilisation and the impact on her identity and Sarah's phantom pregnancy immediately preceding her hysterectomy. In addition to this, encounters with GPs, admission to hospital and the NHS as an institution proved troublesome to women in this study due to the inequalities of power balance. An 'us' and 'them' imagery pervaded the accounts and this was illustrated by stories of dissatisfaction with treatment and lack of communication with the health institution with strong imagery attached. This imagery acts as a metaphor in the accounts by linking the personal to the interpersonal and, in the absence of appropriate narrative to understand and explore the power dynamics, provides a route of explanation and expression of this dissatisfaction. In this study the crisis in identity caused by this power inequality, described by Lisa as 'battling the forces' causes narrative wreckage (Frank, 2000a). The lack of interpersonal relationships available between the person experiencing health and the health institution is a key consideration for the women in this study seeking health information and often forced them to look elsewhere for knowledge. The participants reported that alternative health solutions such as homeopathy provided a more relational route to solving health problems, as did searching the internet and finding other mediated sources of information. This suggests that, although the women were generally unaware of the implicit power inequality present in institutionalised health due to its objectification of women through Cartesian dualism, they will, due to their holistic monitoring of their health status and stoical attitude, take action to step outside the patriarchal medical model of health and look elsewhere for a solution. Paula Kamen argues that:

> A natural response is to change the word feminist to a word with fewer stigmas attached. But inevitably the same thing will happen to that magical word. Part of the radical connotation of feminism is not due to the word, but to the action. The act of a woman standing up for herself is radical, whether she calls herself a feminist or not. (Kamen, 1991, p.56)

This, along with the action of volunteering for this study, suggests that feminist action is taken to solve these health problems. This supports Butler's (1990) feminist model of gender politics, where gender is performed in society and is relational to the psychosocio-cultural aspects of the individual woman's life. In this study, the women live in deprived economic conditions, both personally and in the general community. As a result of living in an area that has long been economically deprived, they are more at risk of educational deprivation and health provision inequality. This combination of social deprivation leaves these women disempowered, and at an opposite end of the power dialectic from the hegemonic institutionalised health system. Further, their awareness of feminist action is limited to the stigmatised version of second wave feminism which endorses radical action (Harstock, 1999). In addition to this, their perceptions of family are around the idealised traditional family, with the man as the head of the family (Coser, 1977), and in many cases in this study this is not the case, causing additional identity conflict. However, these women are implicitly aware of their disempowerment and although they do not express their views in clear political terms, they go some way to address the move along the power dialectic by their strength in adversity and their expression of their dissatisfaction with the medical model of health. The construction, reconstruction and performance of their health identity in the light of impending fertility is an example of gender politics (Butler, 1990), as these women individually move towards a satisfactory health identity by re-negotiating their health knowledge. This identity construction represents a synthesis between the powerlessness the women feel and the power they feel institutionalised health holds. These complex health considerations, both implicit and explicit run through the narrative accounts and themes of holistic health that emerged and provide an interactive model of the construction of health identity, as shown in Figure 9.1.

These interactive levels, however, do not generalise the health experience. Although the women in the study are experiencing peri-menopausal health identity, their stories have very different life trajectories (Frank, 2000a) due to the unique nature of individual, social

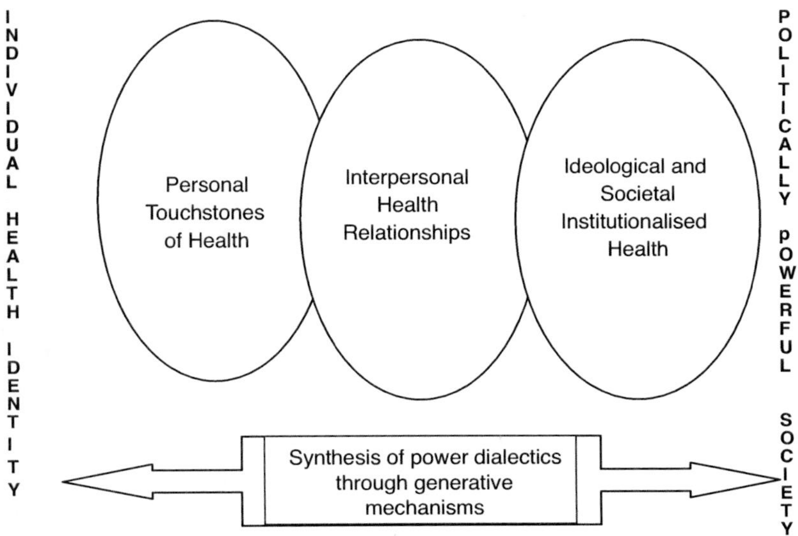


*Figure 9.1* An integrated explanatory model of health identity construction

and cultural experiences. The personal layer of fragmented health identity is the personal story of perimenopausal health that forms the chronological basis of the narrative account. The interpersonal layer of fragmented health represents the embodiment of the health experience in the world with others and is multidirectional and interactive with the personal layer. These two layers, in the narratives of interpersonal health, align with each other in the interpersonal accounts of health the women give of experiences with family, friends and healthcare providers. Conflict occurs, however, when the third positional and ideological layer of fragmented health identity is introduced, as this provides women with a confused sense of 'who I am' compared to 'who I should be' according to societal and cultural representations of women's health. This ideological level of identity construction emphasises that different health 'truths' are available to women and that the various ideologies within this level are further fragmented. Together, these layers form a negotiated synthesis of identity construction that attempts to resolve the dialectical-political positions of power between the individual and society.

The material body has been problematic for feminist theory and a lot of theory has focused on social constructs of feminism in gender performance (Bulter, 1990) and standpoint theory (Harding, 1996) that focuses on social expression of feminism. Whilst this is important and valid, the body must be combined into theory to encompass the inclusion of material consideration of health identity, which, in this study, was represented by the emplotment of the narrative accounts being based on physical reproductive health milestones.

These realist assumptions have been used in this book to illustrate the material body and infradian rhythmic cycles that underlie reproductive health and relativist assumptions of lived social experience that include personal, interpersonal and institutionalised health experiences. The closed system of intransive reality acknowledges the importance of the medical model for the material body. The open systems of transive relativism operate on two levels, the empirical domain where theory resides and the deep domain where epistemic operations take place. Although the model below deconstructs these levels and domains, this study has shown that health identity is a constantly fluid and flexible process which constructs and reconstructs itself on the basis of all these levels of philosophical considerations. Therefore, the process of constructing the health identity is important as this shows how the health identity, as opposed to what, is constructed.

In this study, the embodiment of health identity was expressed in the narrative accounts by the women who took part. However, the

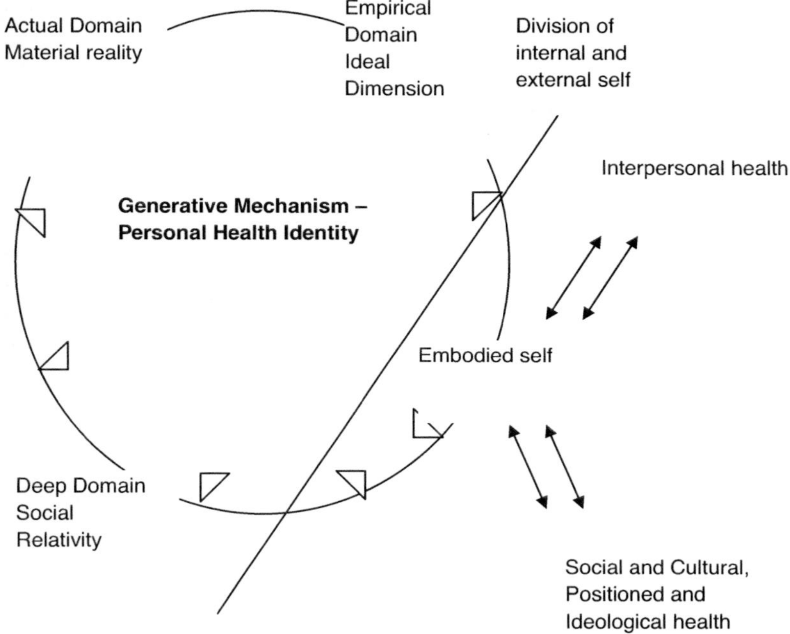


*Figure 9.2* A model of the generative mechanisms of the construction of health identity

dialectical embodiment of health identity in society was seen in terms of interpersonal relationships and in the mediation of health through society. Because of the multidirectional nature of the embodiment of health, and the fluidity of health identity, certain interventions would be possible to improve the health experience for women.

## Identity actions

The theoretical aspects of this work and the rich, detailed accounts of the women have provided a collaboration of abstract and solid work underpinning a model of identity construction. However, the application of such a model in real-life terms is important if we are to understand how identity works everyday. The analysis of the accounts in terms of identity actions as opposed to further labelling and stereotyping women in terms of pre-conceived concepts provides the work with flexibility. The fluid nature of identity construction discussed in Chapter 3 is mapped onto everyday lived experience through the use of evolving concepts which themselves are flexible and mutable. It is at this point this story of identity construction ends, with a psychological and philosophical positioning of identity in a model which both expresses and frees the accounts of the women who took part in this study.

## Concluding comments

The study that this work is based upon clearly has limitations. While the research was based on a sample of women from a disadvantaged area and represented the ethnic differences in the proportion to which they occur in this area, the sample was relatively small. This project, in this sense, is a starting point where the health identities of these women within the context of their whole lives and lived experience. At the beginning of this project it was informally theorised that the information given in the interviews would be mainly pertaining to health, but as the work continued it became clear that the narrative accounts of the women would be a portrait of their lives, a mixed landscape from which the health identity would need to be carefully highlighted.

The work was intricate and time consuming at times and constantly threw up new challenges of reflexive thinking. Although the sample was small, the amount of information rich data obtained both formally in interviews and informally in briefing sessions and meetings was huge and wide ranging. It soon became clear that, compared with current health facilities and government planning for health, these women were often organising their own health outside institutionalised models. This required a person-centred modelling of health identity and therefore a deeper philosophical approach to this modelling which was found in the critical realist approach to health.

Contemplating the scale of the complexities of how women construct their health identities was a major task and the findings from the interview study expanded the original expectation of the sources for which the identity was constructed, particularly across overlapping issues such as pre-menstrual syndrome and the menopause. This, in turn, highlighted the explanatory language used by health professionals and some academics to group together and define (and sometimes stereotype) different types of health problems away from everyday lived experience. The development of the use of identity actions in this study brings a flexibility and fluidity to identity construction that cannot be highlighted enough. After all, each woman in the study brought her own individual story crafted from her own individual experience that continued to flow, even through the course of the project, and change.

In terms of the feminist underpinning to this project, the women both struggled and coped with health, depending on the health relationships. Most had a firm personal idea of what health was and how to maintain it, yet this was often confounded by the Cartesian dualistic aspects of institutionalised health and how this is represented through society. Whilst none of the women who were interviewed stated explicitly that they were feminist the narrative accounts suggest that, at least at a personal level, they feel empowered to make their own choices about how they obtain information about health. It is at the point of service, the hospital, the GP, the media, even organised institutions such as church and family, that they begin to feel disempowered. However, this was rarely due to individual relationships, rather with an institutionalised 'them and us' construction of health power dynamics.

The models in this book were developed both as an explanation of the complexities of this study and as guidelines for future studies into identity construction. The development of a set model is not ideal when considering a project which starts at the unique personal level and expands to an institutional level. The conflicts between the unique and the general in the methodology were eased with the qualitative understanding that this study, like identity, is flexible and evolving. Therefore, it would be hoped that the models developed, particularly Figure 8.1 which identifies the identity actions in this project, could be used as a template for study in all areas of identity construction. Along with the critical realist model and the connections between personal, interpersonal and institutionalised health, the modelling creates a multidimensional template for the study of identity; the aim of this is so as to not disempower by fixed values and labelling and indeed a definition of a single identity based on a simple analysis of those aspects of a person that are most obvious over a short time, or single areas of study.

Finally, some of the women who took part in this study have read the work that evolved from it and one of them commented thus:

> This is great. I'm a person, not a number. Now I've said what I wanted to say for ages. (Michelle, debriefing)

Although this may seem obvious and a given to many, for her it meant a break away from objectification and empowerment toward voice. It would be difficult to find a more convincing case for qualitative, narrative methodology and a critical approach to inequality and injustice than this.

# References

Adams, T. (2000). 'The discursive construction of identity by community psychiatric nurses and family members caring for people with dementia'. *Journal of Advanced Nursing*, Vol 32 (4): 791–798.

Al-Azzawi (1991). 'Endrocrinology aspects of menopause'. *British Medical Bulletin*, Vol 48 (2): 262.

Alex, L. (2004). 'Women's experiences in connection with induced abortion – A feminist perspective'. *Nordic College of Caring Sciences*, Vol 18: 160–168.

Alexander, F. (1950). *Psychosomatic Medicine*. New York: Norton.

Anderson, A.S., Cox, D.N., McKellar, S., Reynolds, J., Lean, M.E.J. & Mela, D.J. (1998). 'Take five, a nutrition education intervention to increase fruit and vegetable intakes: Impact on attitudes towards dietary change'. *British Journal of Nutrition*, Vol 80 (2): 133–140.

Andrews, M., Squire, C. and Tamboukou, M. (2008) *Doing Narrative Research*. London: Sage.

Bakhtin, M.M. (1981). *The Dialogic Imagination: Four Essays by M.M. Bakhtin* (M. Holquist (ed.); C. Emerson & M. Holquist, Trans.). Austin: University of Texas Press.

Banister, P., Burman, E., Parker, I., Taylor, M. & Tindall, C. (1998). *Qualitative Methods in Psychology – A Research Guide*. Buckingham: OU Press.

Barbre, J. (1998). 'Meno-boomers and moral guardians: An exploration of the cultural construction of menopause'. In Weitz, R. (ed.) *The Politics of Women's Bodies: Sexuality Appearance and Behavior*, pp.163–178. New York: Oxford University Press.

Barker, D.K. (1999). 'Emancipatory for whom? A comment of critical realism'. *Feminist Economics*, Vol 9 (1): 103–108.

Bartky, S. (1998) 'Foucalt, femininity, and the modernization of patriarchal power'. In Kournay, J.A., Sterba, J.J., Tong, R.R. & Cliffs, E. (eds) *Feminist Philosophies: Problems, Theories and Applications*. NJ: Prentice Hall.

Bartlett, F.C. (1932). *Remembering*. Cambridge: Cambridge University Press.

Baum, A. (1999). 'Health psychology: Mapping biobehavioural contributions to health and illness'. *Annual Review of Psychology 1999*.

Bhaskar, R. (1978). *A Realist Theory of Science*. Hassocks: Harvester Press.

Blumler, J.G. & Katz, E. (1974). *The Uses of Mass Communication*. Newbury Park, CA: Sage.

Bolam, B. & Chaimberlain, K. (2003). 'Professionalization and reflexivity in critical health psychology practice'. *Journal of Health Psychology*, Vol 8 (2): 215–218.

Bolam, B., Gleeson, K. & Murphy, S. (2003). '"Lay person" or "health expert"? exploring theoretical and practical aspects of reflexivity in qualitative health research'. *Forum: Qualitative Social Research*, Vol 4 (2).

Boneham, M.A. & Sixsmith, J.A. (2005). 'The voices of older women in a disadvantaged community: Issues of health and social capital'. *Social Science and Medicine*, Vol 62: 269–279.

Bonner, F., Goodman, L., Allen, R., Janes, L. & King, K. (1992). *Imagining Women: Cultural Representations and Gender*. Cambridge: Polity Press.

Bowles, C.L. (1990). 'The menopausal experience: Sociocultural influences and theoretical models'. In Formanek, R. (ed.) *The Meanings of Menopause: Historical, Medical and Clinical Perspectives*, pp.157–177. Hilsdale, NJ: Analytic Press.

Bridgens, R. (2004). 'Walking and work: Narratives of polio and postpolio syndrome'. In Kelly, N., Horrocks, C., Milnes, K., Roberts, B. & Robinson, D. (eds) *Narrative Memory and Everyday Life*, pp.125–135. Huddersfield: University of Huddersfield.

British Psychological Society (BPS) (1978). 'Ethical principles for research with human subjects'. *Bulletin of the British Psychological Society*, Vol 31: 48–49.

British Psychological Society (BPS) (2000). *Code of Conduct, Ethical Principles and Guidelines*. Leicester: British Psychological Society.

Burger, H.G., Dudley, E.C., Robertson, D.M. & Dennerstein, L. (2002). 'Hormonal changes in the menopause transition'. *Recent Progress in Hormone Research*, Vol 57: 257–275.

Burkitt, I. (1998). *Social Selves: Theories of the Social Formation of the Personality*. London: Sage.

Burkitt, I. (2004). 'Biography and narrative in the times and places of everyday life'. In Kelly, N., Horrocks, C., Milnes, K., Roberts, B. & Robinson, D. (eds) *Narrative Memory and Everyday Life*, pp.69–87. Huddersfield: University of Huddersfield.

Butler, J. (1990). *Gender Trouble*. London: Routledge.

Chater, K. (2002). 'Ageing: A body of resistance'. *Nursing and Health Sciences*, Vol 4: 123–129.

Chomsky, N. (1989). 'Some notes on the economy of derivation and representation'. In Freidin, R. (ed.) *Principles and Parameters in Comparative Grammar*. Cambridge, MA: MIT Press.

Christodoulou, J.A. (2006). 'An autobiography of health: The story so far'. In Milnes, K., Horrocks, C., Kelly, N., Roberts, B. & Robinson, D. (eds) *Narrative, Memory and Knowledge: Representations, Aesthetics and Context*, pp.127–135. Huddersfield: University of Huddersfield.

Clinckinbeard, C., Minton, B.A., Davis, J. and McDermott, K. (1999). 'Women's knowledge about menopause, hormone replacement therapy (HRT) and interactions with healthcare providers: An exploratory study'. *Journal of Women's Health & Gender Based Medicine*, Vol 8 (8): 1097–1011.

Collins, K. & Nicolson, P. (2002). 'The meaning of "satisfaction" for people with dermatological problems: Re-assessing approaches to qualitative health psychology research'. *Journal of Health Psychology*, Vol 7 (5): 615–629.

Conboy, K., Medina, N. & Stanbury, S. (1997). *Writing on the Body: Female Embodiment and Feminist Theory*. New York: Columbia University Press.

Coser, L.A. (1977). *Masters of Sociological Thought: Ideas in Historical and Social Context*. Second edition. New York: Harcourt Brace Jovanovich.

Courtenay, W.H. (2000). 'Constructions of masculinity and their influence on men's well-being: A theory of gender and health'. *Social Science and Medicine*, Vol 50: 1385–1401.

Crossley, M.L. (1998). 'Sick role or empowerment: The ambiguities of life with a HIV-positive diagnosis'. *Sociology of Health and Illness*, Vol 20 (4): 507–531.

Crossley, M.L. (2000a). *Rethinking Health Psychology*. Buckingham: Open University Press.

Crossley, M.L. (2000b). *Introducing Narrative Psychology: Self, Trauma and the Construction of Meaning*. Buckingham: Open University Press.

Crowley, H. & Himmelweit, S. (1992). *Knowing Women: Feminism and Knowledge*. Cambridge: Polity Press.

Cuevas, C.D. & Sanz, E.J. (2006). 'Safety of selective serotonin reuptake inhibitors in pregnancy'. *Current Drug Safety,* Vol 1 (1): 17–24.

Cussins, A.M. (2001). 'The role of body image in women's mental health'. *Feminist Review,* Vol 68: 105–114.

Danermark, B., Ekstrom, M., Jakobsen, L. & Karlson, J.C. (2002). *Explaining Society – Critical Realism in the Social Science*. London: Routledge.

Darwin, C. (1859). *On the Origin of the Species by Means of Natural Selection*. Murray.

Dawkins, R. (1993). *The Selfish Gene*. Oxford: Oxford University Press.

De Beauvoir, S. (1949). *The Second Sex*. London: Random House.

Dell, D.L. & Stewart, D.E. (2000). 'Menopause and mood: Is depression linked with hormone changes?', *Postgrad Med,* Vol 108 (3): 39–43.

Denious, J. & Russo, N.F. (2000). 'The socio-political context of abortion and its relationship to women's mental health'. In Ussher, J.M. (ed.) *Women's Health*. London: BPS.

Descartes, R. (1647). 'Meditationes de prima philosophia, in qua dei existentia et animae immortalitas demonstratur'. In Lafluer, L. (ed.) *Discourse on Method and the Meditations: 1969 Translation*. Harmondsworth: Penguin.

Dhiman, R.K. & Chawlw, Y.K. (2006). 'Is there a link between oestrogen therapy and gallbladder disease?'. *Expert Opinion on Drug Safety,* Vol 5 (1): 117–129.

Doise, W. (1986). 'Les représentations sociales: Définition d'un concept'. In Doise, W. & Palmonari, A. (eds) *L'étude des représentations sociales,* pp.81–94. Paris: Delachaux et Niestle.

Dunbar, F. (1943). *Psychosomatic Diagnosis*. New York: Hoeber.

Duncan, B.L. (1979). 'The effects of race of harm-doer and victim on social perception and attributional behaviour'. *Journal of Psychology,* Vol 101: 103–105.

Easton, K.L., McComish, J.F. & Greenberg, R. (2000). 'Avoiding common pitfalls in qualitative research'. *Qualitative Health Research,* Vol 10 (5): 703–707.

Engel, G.L. (1977). 'The clinical application of the biopsychosocial model'. *American Journal of Psychiatry,* Vol 137: 535–544.

Etherington, K. (2004). *Becoming a Reflexive Researcher – Using Our Selves in Research*. London: Kingsley.

Fauconnier, A., Ringa, V., Delanoe, D., Falissard, B. & Breart, G. (2000). 'Use of hormone replacement therapy: Women's representations of menopause and beauty care practices'. *Maturitas,* Vol 35: 215–228.

Fergusson, D.M., Horwood, L.J. & Ridder, E.M. (2006). 'Abortion in young women and subsequent mental health'. *Journal of Child Psychology and Psychiatry,* Vol 47 (1): 16–24.

Fishbein, M. & Yzer, M.C. (2003). 'Using theory to design effective health behaviour interventions'. *Communication Theory,* Vol 13 (2): 164–183.

Foucault, M. (1978). *The Will to Knowledge: The History of Sexuality Part 1*. Middlesex: Penguin.

Fox Keller, E. (1984). *Untitled Article in Technology Review,* Vol 87 (8): 45–47.

Francis, B. (2002). 'Relativism, realism and feminism: An analysis of some theoretical research on gender identity'. *Journal of Gender Studies,* Vol 11 (1): 39–54.

Frank, A.W. (2000a). *The Wounded Storyteller*. Chicago: Chicago University Press.

Frank, A.W. (2000b). 'The standpoint of the storyteller'. *Qualitative Health Research,* Vol 10 (3): 354–365.

Fromm, E. (1957) *The Art of Loving*. London: Allen and Unwin.
Gannon, L. & Ekstrom, B. (1993). 'Attitudes towards menopause'. *Psychology of Women Quarterly*, Vol 17: 275–288.
Gannon, L. & Stevens, J. (1998). 'Portraits of menopause in the mass media'. *Women & Health*, Vol 27 (3): 1–15.
Gatchel, J., Baum, A., & Krantz, D.S. (1989). *An Introduction to Health Psychology*. New York: McGraw Books.
Geertz, C. (1973). *Thick Description: Toward an Interpretative Theory of Culture*. NY: Basic Books.
Gergen, K.J. & Davis, K.E. (1985). *The Social Construction of the Person*. New York: Springer.
Gergen, K.J. (1991). *The Saturated Self*. New York: Basic Books.
Gergen, K.J. (1996). 'Psychological science in cultural context'. *American Psychologist*, Vol 51: 496–503.
Gergen, K.J. (1999). 'Social construction and the transformation of identity politics'. In Newmen, F. & Holzman, L. (eds) *End of Knowing: A New Developmental Way of Learning*. New York: Routledge.
Giddens, A. (1991). *Modernity and Self-Identity: Self and Society in the Late Modern Age*. Cambridge: Polity.
Ginev, D. (1998). 'Rhetoric and double hermeneutics in the human sciences'. *Human Studies*, Vol 21 (3): 259–271.
Goffman, E. (1959). *The Presentation of the Self in Everyday Life*. New York: Doubleday Anchor.
Goldberg, L. (2002). 'Rethinking the birthing body: Cartesian dualism and perinatal nursing'. *Journal of Advanced Nursing*, Vol 37 (5): 446–451.
Gramsci, A. (1971). *Selections from Prison Notebooks*. New York: International Publishers.
Greene, S. (2000). 'Choosing a life span developmental orientation'. In Ussher, J.M. (ed.) *Women's Health*, pp.50–59. London: BPS.
Griffin, C. & Lyons, A. (2000). 'Representations of menopause and women at midlife'. In Ussher, J.M. (ed.) *Women's Health*, pp.470–475. London: BPS.
Griffiths, F. (1999). 'Women's control and choice regarding HRT'. *Social Science and Medicine*, Vol 49: 469–481.
Gross, H. (2000). 'Pregnancy: A healthy state'. In Ussher, J.M. (ed.) *Women's Health*, pp. 296–302. London: BPS.
Hall, S. (1996). 'Cultural studies: Two paradigms'. In Storey, J. (ed.) *Cultural Studies and the Study of Popular Culture*, pp.31–48. London: OU Press.
Hanson, B. (2001). 'Social constructions of femaleness'. *Qualitative Health Research*, Vol 11: 464–476.
Hardin, P.K. (2003). 'Shape-shifting discourses of anorexia nervosa: Reconstituting psychopathology'. *Nursing Inquiry*, Vol 10 (4): 209–217.
Harding, S. (1986). *The Science Question in Feminism*. New York: Cornell University Press.
Harding, S. (1996). 'Standpoint epistemology (a feminist version): How social disadvantage creates epistemic advantage'. In Turner, S. (ed.) *Social Theory and Sociology: The Classics and Beyond*, pp.146–160. Oxford: Blackwell.
Hardy, R., Kuh, D. & Wadsworth, M. (1999). 'Reproductive characteristics and the age at inception of the perimenopause in a British national cohort'. *International Journal of Epidemiology*, Vol 14 (9): 612–620.

Hardy, R., Kuh, D. & Wadsworth, M. (2000). 'Smoking, body mass index, socio-economic status and the menopausal transition in a British national cohort'. *International Journal of Epidemiology*, Vol 29 (5): 845–851.

Harraway, D.J. (1991). *Simians, Cyborgs and Women: The Reinvention of Nature*. London: Free Association Books.

Harre, R. (1970). *The Principles of Scientific Thinking*. London: Macmillan.

Harre, R. (1983). *Personal Being*. Oxford: Blackwell.

Harre, R. (1992). 'What is real in psychology?'. *Theory and Psychology*, Vol 2 (2): 153–158.

Harre, R. (1994). *The Discursive Mind*. Thousand Oaks: Sage.

Harre, R. (2002). 'Social construction and consciousness'. In Velmans, M. (ed.) *Consciousness*. London: Goldsmiths College.

Harstock, N. (1999). *The Feminist Standpoint Revisited and Other Essays*. New York: Westview Press.

Hennessey, R. (1995). 'Women's lives/feminist knowledge: Feminist standpoint as ideology critique'. Internet resource: Materialist Feminist Archives. http://csr.colorado.edu.mail.matfem/95/0337.html

Hudson, T. (2002). *Perimenopause Naturally – A Friend Indeed*. New York: AFIP.

Indices of Deprivation (2004) http://www.communities.gov.uk/archived/general-content/communities/indicesofdeprivation/216309/

IMD (2004). Department of Environment Transport and the Regions Indices of Deprivation.

Jacobs, P.A., Hyland, M.E. & Ley, A. (2000). 'Self-rated menopausal status and quality of life in women aged 40–63 years'. *British Journal of Health Psychology*, Vol 5 (3): 39–411.

James, W. (1890) (reprinted in 1950). *The Principles of Psychology*. New York: Holt.

John, J.H. & Ziebland, S. (2004). 'Reported barriers to eating more fruit and vegetables before and after participation in a randomized controlled trial: A qualitative study'. *Health Education Research*, Vol 19 (2): 165–174.

Jose, J. (1995). 'Ontological commitment and the concepts of "embodiment" and "embodied person": Some problems for feminist theory'. *Women and Politics*, Vol 15 (1): 19–36.

Kamen, P. (1991). *Feminist Fatale*. New York: Routledge.

Kaufert, P.A. & Lock, M. (1997). 'Medicalisation of women's third age'. *Journal of Psychosomatic Obstetric Gynaecology*, Vol 18: 81–86.

Kelly, C.N.M. & Stanner, S.A. (2003). 'Diet and cardiovascular disease in the UK: Are the messages getting across?'. *Proceedings of the Nutrition Society*, Vol 62 (3): 583–589.

Kim, M. (1997). 'Poor women survey poor women: Feminist perspectives in survey research'. *Feminist Economics*, Vol 3 (2): 99–117.

King, M. & Watson, K. (2005). *Representing Health: Discourses of Health and Illness in the Media*. Hampshire: Palgrave Macmillan.

Kirkham, A. (2001). 'Productive readings: The portrayal of health "experts" in women's magazines'. *Qualitative Health Research*, Vol 11 (6): 751–765.

Komesaroff, P., Rothfield, P. & Daly, J. (1997). *Reinterpreting Menopause: Cultural and Philosophical Issues*. London: Routledge.

Larson, C.L. (1997). 'Re-presenting the subject: Problems in personal narrative enquiry'. *Qualitative Studies in Education*, Vol 10 (4): 455–470.

Lawlor, D.A., Whincup, P., Emberson, J.R., Rees, K., Walker, M. & Ebrahim, S. (2004). 'The challenge of secondary prevention for coronary heart disease in older patients: Findings from the British Women's Heart and Health Study and the British Regional Heart Study'. *Family Practice*, Vol 21 (5): 582–586.

Lawthom, R. (2000). 'Women, stress and work: Exploring the boundaries'. In Ussher, J.M. (ed.) *Women's Health*, pp.423–431. London: BPS.

Lee, C. & Owens, R.G. (2002). 'Issues for a psychology of men's health'. *Journal of Health Psychology*, Vol 7 (3): 209–217.

Lees, S. (2000). 'Sexual assault and domestic violence: Implications for health workers'. In Ussher, J.M. (ed.) *Women's Health*. London: BPS.

Leung, L. (2003). 'Impacts of net-generation attributes, seductive properties of the internet, and gratifications obtained on internet use'. *Telematics and Informatics*, Vol 20 (2): 107–129.

Lock, M. (1998). 'Menopause: Lessons from anthropology'. *Psychosomatic Medicine*, Vol 60: 410–419.

Luff, D. (1999). 'Dialogue across the divides: Moments of rapport and power in feminist research with anti-feminist women'. *Sociology*, Vol 33 (4): 687–703.

Luksha, L. & Kublickiene, K. (2005). 'Implications for endothelium-derived hyperpolarising factor (EDHF) in women's cardiovascular health'. *Current Women's Health Reviews*, Vol 1 (1): 67–78.

Lyon, M. (1996). 'Wright Mills meets Prozac: The relevance of "social emotion" to the sociology of health and illness'. In James, V. and Gabe, J. (eds) *Health and the Sociology of Emotion*. Oxford: Blackwell.

Lyons, A.C (2000). 'Examining media representations: Benefits for health psychology'. *Journal of Health Psychology*, Vol 5 (3): 349–358.

Lyons, A. & Griffin, C. (2002). 'Managing menopause: A qualitative study of self-help literature for women at midlife'. *Social Science and Medicine*, Vol 56 (8): 1629–1642.

Malos, E. (1995). *The Politics of Housework*. Padstow: T.J. Press.

Marks, D., Murray, M., Evans, B., Willig, C., Sykes, A.M. & Woodall, C. (2001). *Health Psychology: Theory, Research and Practice*. London: Sage.

Martsolf, D.S. & Mickley, J.R. (1998). 'The concept of spirituality in nursing theories: Differing world-views and extent of focus'. *Journal of Advanced Nursing*, Vol 27: 294–303.

Martin, V.T. & Behbehani, M. (2006). 'Ovarian hormones and migraine headache: Understanding mechanisms and pathogenesis'. *Headache: The Journal of Head and Face Pain*, Vol 46 (1): 3–23.

Marx, K. (1954). *Capital? Volume I*. London: Lawrence & Wishart.

Maslow, A.H. (1965). *Eupsychian Management – A Journal*. Homewood: Irwin.

Maslow, A.H. (1968). *Towards a Psychology of Being*. Princeton NJ: Von Nostrand.

May, R. (1983). *The Discovery of Being: Writings in Existential Psychology*. London: W.W. Norton.

May, V. (2004). 'Narrative identity and the re-conceptualisation of lone motherhood'. *Narrative Inquiry*, Vol 16: 305–315.

McAdams, D.P. (1993). *The Stories We Live By: Personal Myths and the Making of the Self*. New York: William Morrow and Co.

Mead, G.H. (1934). *Mind, Self and Society*. Chicago: University of Chicago Press.

Mearleau-Ponty, M. (1945). *Phenomenology of Perception*. Paris: Gallimard.

Mercer, K. (1990). 'Welcome to the jungle'. In Rutherford, J. (ed.) *Identity: Community, Culture, Difference*. London: Lawrence & Wishart.

Metcalfe, J. (2000). *The Brain: Degeneration, Damage and Disorder*. New York: Springer-Verlag.

Millgram, S. (1963). 'Behavioural study of obedience'. *Journal of Abnormal and Social Psychology*, Vol 67: 371–378.

Mishler, E.G. (1984). *The Discourse of Medicine: Dialectics of Medical Interview*. New Jersey: Ablex.

Mishler, E.G. (1995). 'Models of narrative analysis: A typology'. *The Journal of Narrative and Life History*, Vol 5 (2): 87–123.

Mishler, E.G. (1999). *Storylines: Craftartists' Narratives of Identity*. Massachusetts: Harvard University Press.

Misri, S. & Kendrick, K. (2006). 'Paroxetine use in the treatment of premenstrual dysmorphic disorder'. *Women's Health*, Vol 2 (1): 43–51.

Morse, C. (2000). 'Reproduction: A critical analysis'. In Ussher, J.M. (ed.) *Women's Health*, pp.290–296. London: BPS.

Moscovici, S. (1984). 'The phenomenon of social representations'. In Farr, R.M. & Moscovici, S. (eds) *Social Representations*. Cambridge: Cambridge University Press.

Murray, M. (2000). 'Levels of narrative analysis in health psychology'. *Journal of Health Psychology*, Vol 5 (3): 337–347.

Murray, M. & Campbell, C. (2003). 'Living in a material world'. *Journal of Health Psychology*, Vol 8 (2): 231–236.

Murray, R.B. & Zentner, J.P. (1989). *Nursing Concepts for Health Promotion*. London: Prentice Hall.

Murtagh, M. & Hepworth, J. (2003). 'Menopause as a long-term risk to health: Implications of general practitioner accounts of prevention for women's choice and decision-making'. *Sociology of Health and Illness*, Vol 25 (2): 185–207.

NHS Website (2007) http://www.nhs.uk/NHSEngland/thenhs/about/Pages/overview.aspx

O'Sullivan, T., Dutton, B. & Rayner, P. (1994). *Studying the Media*. London: Hodder Arnold.

Oakley, A. (1981). 'Interviewing women: A contradiction in terms'. In Roberts, H. (ed.) *Doing Feminist Research*. New York: Routledge.

Oedegaard, K.J., Neckelmann, A., Dahl, A., Zwart, J., Hagen, K. & Fasmer, O. (2006). 'Migraine with and without aura: Association with depression and anxiety disorder in a population-based study: The Hunt Study'. *Cephalalgia*, Vol 26 (1): 1–6.

Ogden, J. (2000). *Health Psychology – A Textbook*. Buckinghamshire: OU Press.

Popay, J. (1992). 'My health is all right, but I'm just tired all the time'. In Roberts, H. (ed.) *Women's Health Matters*, pp.99–120. London: Routledge.

Popay, J., Thomas, C., Williams, G., Bennett, S., Gatrell, A. & Bostock, L. (2003). 'A proper place to live: Health inequalities, agency and the normative dimensions of space'. *Social Science and Medicine*, Vol 57 (1): 55–69.

Potter, J. & Wetherell, M. (1987). *Discourse and Social Psychology: Beyond Attitudes and Behaviour*. London: Sage.

Prilleltensky, I. (2005). 'Promoting well-being: Time for a paradigm shift in health and human services'. *Scandinavian Journal of Public Health*, Vol 33 (66): 53–60.

Prilleltensky, I. & Fox, D. (1997). *Critical Psychology*. London: Sage.

Prilleltensky, I. and Nelson, G. (2002). *Doing Psychology Critically: Making a Difference in Diverse Settings*. New York: Macmillan Press.

Public Health Report (2004). Oldham Primary Care Trust.

Radley, A. (2000). 'Health psychology, embodiment and the question of vulnerability'. *Journal of Health Psychology*, Vol 5 (3): 297–304.

Ramondetta, L.M. & Sills, D. (2004). 'Spirituality in gynaecological oncology: A review'. *International Journal of Gynaecological Cancer*, Vol 14: 183–201.

Ratner, C. (2002). 'Subjectivity and objectivity in qualitative methodology'. *Forum: Qualitative Social Research*, Vol 3 (3): 67–84.

Reilly, J. (2000). 'PMS research: Balancing the personal and the political'. In Ussher, J.M. (eds) *Women's Health*, pp.255–271. London: BPS.

Ricoeur, P. (1983). *Time and Narrative Volume 1*. Chicago: University Press of Chicago.

Ricoeur, P. (1984). *Time and Narrative Volume 2*. Chicago: University Press of Chicago.

Ricoeur, P. (1985). *Time and Narrative Volume 3*. Chicago: University Press of Chicago.

Ritchie, D. (2001). Oldham independent review report: Oldham Independent Review Panel.

Roberts, B. (2003). 'Life lines, life comments and life traces/forms'. In Robinson, D. (ed.) *Narrative, Memory and Identity: Theoretical and Methodological Issues*. Huddersfield: University of Huddersfield.

Roberts, C. (2000). 'Sex hormones as biocultural actors: Rethinking biology, sexual differences and health'. In Ussher, J.M. (ed.) *Women's Health*, pp.283–290. London: BPS.

Robertson, S. (2007). 'Understanding men and health: Masculinities, identity and well-being'. Berkshire: Open University Press.

Rogers, C.R. (1951). *Client-Centred Therapy*. New York: Houghton.

Ross, L. (2006) 'Spiritual care in nursing: A review of the research to date'. *Journal of Clinical Nursing*, Vol 15 (7): 852–862.

Rostosky, S.S. & Travis, C.B. (1996). 'Menopause research and the dominance of the biomedical model, 1984–1994'. *Psychology of Women Quarterly*, Vol 20: 285–312.

Rudman, L.A. & Glick, P. (2001). 'Prescriptive gender stereotypes and backlash towards agentic women'. *Journal of Social Issues*, Vol 57 (4): 743–762.

Russo, N.F. & Denious, J.E. (1998). 'Why is abortion such a controversial issue in the United States?'. In Beckman, L.J. and Harvey, S.M. (eds) *The New Civil War: The Psychology, Culture, and Politics of Abortion*, pp.25–59. Washington, DC: American Psychological Association.

Samisoe, G. (2002). 'Bleeding problems in middle aged women'. *Maturitas: The European Menopause Journal*, Vol 43 (1): 27–33.

Sapsford, R. (1987). *Issues for Social Psychology*. Milton Keynes: Open University Press.

Sarbin, T.R. (ed.) (1986). *Narrative Psychology: The Storied Nature of Human Conduct*. New York: Preager.

Sayer, A. (2000). *Realism and Social Science*. London: Sage.

Shotter, J. (1997). 'The social construction of our "inner" lives'. *Journal of Constructivist Psychology*, Vol 10: 7–24.

Siega-Riz, A.M., Kelly, R. & Dole, N. (2005). 'Pregnancy related weight gain – A link to obesity'. *Nutrition Reviews*, Vol 1: 105–111.

Sixsmith, J. & Boneham, M. (2003). 'Narrating women's health identities in the context of community living'. In Robinson, D. (ed.) *Narrative, Memory and Identity: Theoretical and Methodological Issues*. Huddersfield: University of Huddersfield.

Social Issues Research Centre (2001). The choices campaign – Jubilee Women: Fiftysomething Women – Lifestyle and attitudes now and fifty years ago.

Stainton-Rodgers, W. & Stainton-Rogers, R. (2001). *The Psychology of Gender and Sexuality*. Buckingham: OU Press.

Stephens, R. (1996). *Understanding the Self*. London: Sage.

Stephens, S., Budge, R.C. & Carryer, J. (2002). 'What is this thing called hormone replacement therapy? Discursive construction of medication in situated practice'. *Qualitative Health Research*, Vol 12 (3): 347–359.

Stoppard, J.M. (2000). 'Understanding depression in women: Limitations of mainstream approaches and a material-discursive alternative'. In Ussher, J.M. (ed.) *Women's Health*. London: BPS.

Swann, C.J. & Ussher, J.M. (1995). 'A discourse analytic approach to women's experience of premenstrual syndrome'. *Journal of Mental Health*, Vol 4: 359–367.

Swinton, J. (2006). 'Identity and resistance: Why spiritual care needs "enemies"'. *Journal of Clinical Nursing*, Vol 15: 918–928.

Tajfel, H. & Turner, J. (1979). 'An integrative theory of group conflict'. In Austin, W.G. & Worschel, S. (eds) *The Social Psychology of Intergroup Relations*. California: Brooks/Cole.

Tajfel, H. & Wilkes, A. (1963). 'Classification of quantitative judgement'. *British Journal of Psychology*, Vol 54: 101–114.

Tang, N. (2002). 'Interviewer and interviewee relationships between women'. *Sociology*, Vol 36 (3): 703–721.

Taylor, S.E. (1999). *Health Psychology*. New York: McGraw-Hill.

Taylor, S. (2004). 'Identity trouble and place of residence in women's life narratives'. In Kelly, N., Horrocks, C., Milnes, K., Roberts, B. & Robinson, D. (eds) *Narrative Memory and Everyday Life*, pp.97–107. Huddersfield: University of Huddersfield.

Thompson, J.K. & Stice, E. (2001). 'Thin-ideal internalisation: Mounting evidence for a new risk factor for body image disturbance and eating pathology'. *American Psychological Society*.

Toates, F. (1998). *Biology, Brain & Behaviour: Control of Behaviour*. New York: Springer-Verlag.

Tolman, D.L. (2000). 'Femininity as a barrier to positive sexual health for adolescent girls'. In Ussher, J.M. (ed.) *Women's Health*, pp.93–105. London: BPS.

Ussher, J.M. (1991). *Women's Madness: Misogyny or Mental Illness?* New York: Harverster Wheatsheaf.

Ussher, J.M. (1997). *Body Talk: The Material and Discursive Regulation of Sexuality, Madness and Reproduction*. New York: Routledge.

Ussher, J.M. (2000). *Women's Health*. London: BPS.

Vanselow, W. (2000). 'What does systems theory have to do with premenstrual complaints?'. In Ussher, J.M. (ed.) *Women's Health*, pp.266–271. London: BPS.

Washington, M. (1993). *Narrative of Sojourner Truth*. New York: Random House.

Weber, M. (1962). *Basic Concepts in Sociology*. New York: The Citadel Press.
Webster, R. (1996). *Why Freud was Wrong: Sin, Science and Psychoanalysis*. Revised edition. London: HarperCollins.
Weitz, R. (1998). *The Politics of Women's Bodies: Sexuality Appearance and Behavior*. New York: Oxford University Press.
Wetherell, M. & Maybin, J. (1996). 'The distributed self: A social constructionist perspective'. In Stevens, J. (ed.) *Understanding the Self*. London: Sage.
Wilcox, K. & Laird, J. (2000). 'The impact of media images of super slender women on women's self-esteem: Identification, social comparison and self-perception'. *Journal of Research in Personality*, Vol 34: 278–286.
Wilde, M.A. (1999). 'Embodiment'. *Journal of Advanced Nursing*, Vol 22 (2): 25–38.
Wilkinson, S. (1996). *Feminist Social Psychologies: International Perspectives*. Guildford: Biddles.
Williams, M.S., Thomsen, S.R. & McCoy, J.K. (2003). 'Looking for an accurate mirror: A model for the relationship between media use and anorexia'. *Eating Behaviours*, Vol 4 (2): 127–134.
Williams, S.J. (1999). 'Is anybody there? Critical realism, chronic illness and the disability debate'. *Sociology of Health and Illness*, Vol 21 (6): 797–819.
Witz, A. (2000). 'Whose body matters? Feminist sociology and the corporeal turn in sociology and feminism'. *Body and Society*, Vol 6 (2): 1–24.
Women's Health Initiative (2002). 'Risks and benefits of estrogen plus progestin in healthy postmenopausal women'. *The Journal of the American Medical Association*, Vol 281: 321–333.
Woodward, K. (2004). *Questioning Identity: Gender, Class, Ethnicity*. London: Routledge, Open University.
Wright, S.G. (2005). *Reflections on Spirituality and Health*. London: Whurr Publishers.
Yardley, L. (1997). *Material Discourses of Health and Illness*. New York: Routledge.
Zigmond, A.S. & Snaith, R.P. (1983). 'The hospital anxiety and depression scale'. *Acta Psychiatricia Scandinavia*, Vol 67: 361–370.

## Contact details for Dr Jacqueline Christodoulou CPsychol

If you would like to contact me regarding this book or other research matters please email me at Social Analysis and Research Services
www.rosics.com
info@rosics.com

## Domestic Violence Helplines

| | |
|---|---|
| Oldham Family Crisis Group | **0161 628 4991** |
| National Domestic Violence Helpline | **0808 2000 247** |

# Index